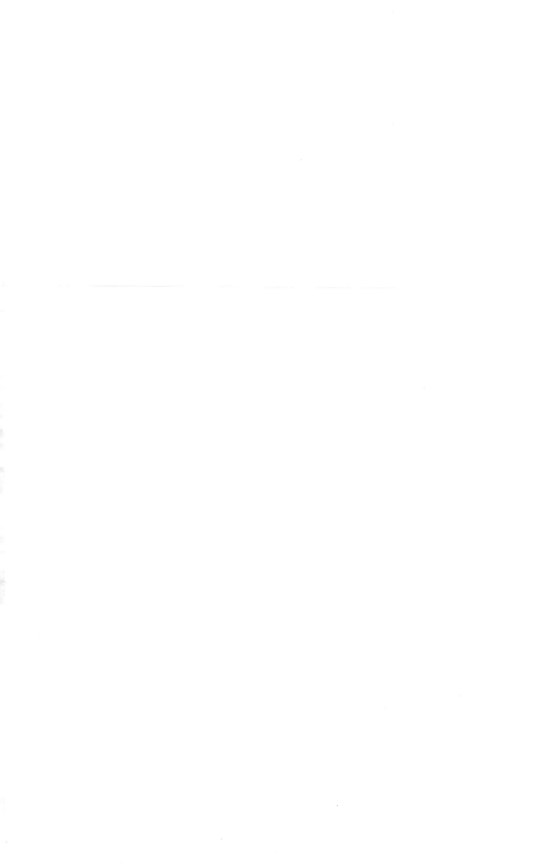

Abdominal Transplantation

Editor

CLAUS U. NIEMANN

ANESTHESIOLOGY CLINICS

www.anesthesiology.theclinics.com

Consulting Editor
LEE FLEISHER

December 2013 • Volume 31 • Number 4

ELSEVIER

1600 John F. Kennedy Boulevard • Suite 1800 • Philadelphia, Pennsylvania, 19103-2899
http://www.theclinics.com

ANESTHESIOLOGY CLINICS Volume 31, Number 4
December 2013 ISSN 1932-2275, ISBN-13: 978-0-323-26086-2

Editor: Jennifer Flynn-Briggs
Developmental Editor: Susan Showalter

Anesthesiology Clinics (ISSN 1932-2275) is published quarterly by Elsevier Inc., 360 Park Avenue South, New York, NY 10010-1710. Months of issue are March, June, September, and December. Periodicals postage paid at New York, NY and at additional mailing offices. Subscription prices are $154.00 per year (US student/resident), $313.00 per year (US individuals), $383.00 per year (Canadian individuals), $516.00 per year (US institutions), $639.00 per year (Canadian institutions), $216.00 per year (Canadian and foreign student/resident), $434.00 per year (foreign individuals), and $639.00 per year (foreign institutions). To receive student and resident rate, orders must be accompanied by name of affiliated institution, date of term, and the *signature* of program/residency coordinator on institutions letterhead. Orders will be billed at individual rate until proof of status is received. Foreign air speed delivery is included in all *Clinics'* subscription prices. All prices are subject to change without notice. POSTMASTER: Send address changes to *Anesthesiology Clinics,* Elsevier Health Sciences Division, Subscription Customer Service, 3251 Riverport Lane, Maryland Heights, MO 63043. Customer Service (orders, claims, online, change of address): Elsevier Health Sciences Division, Subscription Customer Service, 3251 Riverport Lane, Maryland Heights, MO 63043. Tel: 1-800-654-2452 (U.S. and Canada); 314-447-8871 (outside U.S. and Canada). Fax: 314-447-8029. E-mail: journalscustomerservice-usa@elsevier.com (for print support); journalsonlinesupport-usa@elsevier.com (for online support).

Reprints. For copies of 100 or more of articles in this publication, please contact the Commercial Reprints Department, Elsevier Inc., 360 Park Avenue South, New York, NY 10010-1710. Tel.: 212-633-3874; Fax: 212-633-3820; E-mail: reprints@elsevier.com.

Anesthesiology Clinics, is also published in Spanish by McGraw-Hill Inter-americana Editores S. A., P.O. Box 5-237, 06500 Mexico D. F., Mexico.

Anesthesiology Clinics, is covered in *MEDLINE/PubMed (Index Medicus), Current Contents/Clinical Medicine, Excerpta Medica, ISI/BIOMED*, and *Chemical Abstracts*.

Printed and bound by CPI Group (UK) Ltd, Croydon, CR0 4YY

Transferred to digital print 2012

Contributors

CONSULTING EDITOR

LEE A. FLEISHER, MD, FACC, FAHA
Robert D. Dripps Professor and Chair of Anesthesiology and Critical Care, Professor of Medicine, Perelman School of Medicine, University of Pennsylvania School of Medicine, Philadelphia, Pennsylvania

EDITOR

CLAUS U. NIEMANN, MD
Professor of Anesthesia and Surgery, Department of Anesthesia and Perioperative Care; Division of Transplantation, Department of Surgery, University of California San Francisco, San Francisco, California

AUTHORS

T. ANTHONY ANDERSON, MD, PhD
Department of Anesthesia, Massachusetts General Hospital, Harvard Medical School, Boston, Massachusetts

ANTONIA J. CRONIN, MA, PhD, MRCP (UK)
Consultant Nephrologist and Honorary Senior Lecturer, NIHR Biomedical Research Centre, Guy's and St Thomas' NHS Foundation Trust, MRC Centre for Transplantation, Guy's Hospital, King's College London, London, United Kingdom

GERALDINE C. DIAZ, DO
Department of Anesthesia and Critical Care, University of Chicago, Chicago, Illinois

HELGE EILERS, MD
Associate Professor, Anesthesia and Perioperative Care, University of California San Francisco School of Medicine, San Francisco, California

JAMES Y. FINDLAY, MB, ChB, FRCA
Consultant, Department of Anesthesiology and Critical Care Medicine; Assistant Professor, Mayo Clinic College of Medicine, Mayo Clinic, Rochester, Minnesota

LAURA HAMMEL, MD
Assistant Professor of Anesthesiology, University of Wisconsin School of Medicine and Public Health, Madison, Wisconsin

JULIE K. HEIMBACH, MD
Division of Transplantation Surgery, Mayo Clinic, Rochester, Minnesota

ZOLTAN HEVESI, MD, MBA
Professor of Anesthesiology and Surgery, University of Wisconsin School of Medicine and Public Health, Madison, Wisconsin

PRAVEEN KANDULA, MD
Department of Medicine, Massachusetts General Hospital, Harvard Medical School, Boston, Massachusetts

DARREN MALINOSKI, MD, FACS
Associate Professor of Surgery, Portland VA Medical Center, Oregon Health & Science University, Portland, Oregon

MICHAEL RAMSAY, MD, FRCA
Chairman, Department of Anesthesiology and Pain Management, Baylor University Medical Center; President, Baylor Research Institute; Clinical Professor, University of Texas Southwestern Medical School, Dallas Texas

JOHN F. RENZ, MD, PhD
Section of Abdominal Organ Transplantation, Department of Surgery, University of Chicago, Chicago, Illinois

MITCHELL SALLY, MD
Assistant Professor of Surgery, Portland VA Medical Center, Oregon Health & Science University, Portland, Oregon

MICHAEL D. SPIRO, MD
Visiting Assistant Professor, Anesthesia and Perioperative Care, University of California San Francisco School of Medicine, San Francisco, California

PARSIA A. VAGEFI, MD, FACS
Division of Transplant Surgery, Department of Surgery, Massachusetts General Hospital, Harvard Medical School, Boston, Massachusetts

GEBHARD WAGENER, MD
Department of Anesthesiology, Columbia University College of Physicians and Surgeons, New York, New York

Contents

The history of medicine is that what was inconceivable yesterday and barely achievable today often becomes routine tomorrow. Liver transplantation began with almost no resources at the same time as the tentative first steps were taken to land a man on the moon. Because human lives would be at stake, both objectives had a sacramental element from the outset: a solemnly binding commitment to perfection. The gift of an organ is really a gift of life, and something as valuable as a life-saving organ is more important to a suffering patient than wealth or power. The concept of a team approach to the care of the transplant patient is an important factor in the development of a successful program. This has resulted in recipient survival rates reaching 90% at one year.

Organ transplantation has evolved into the standard of care for patients with end-stage organ failure. Despite considering increasingly complex transplant recipients for organs recovered from donors with increasing comorbid conditions, 1-year patient survival following kidney transplantation is 97% in the United States, whereas liver transplant recipient 1-year survival is 90%. There were 16,485 kidney recipients in the United States in 2012, and 6256 patients who underwent liver transplantation. The intent of this review is to highlight the logistics required for transplantation as well as reviewing the current oversight of transplantation.

Over the last 6 decades, organ transplantation has achieved great success to become standard therapy for the treatment of patients with end-stage organ failure. With this success has emerged candidate wait lists that greatly outnumber the current supply of deceased donor organs. The increasing number of candidates and transplants performed has resulted in an organ allocation process that occurs at a local, regional, and sometimes national level. A brief description of the history is presented as well as the methodologies involved in allocation of a donor organ to a single recipient.

Transplantation of nonstandard or expanded criteria donor organs creates several potential ethical and legal problems in terms of consent and liability, and new challenges for research and service development; it highlights the need for a system of organ donation that responds to an evolving ethical landscape and incorporates scientific innovation to meet the needs of recipients, but which also safeguards the interests and autonomy of the donor. In this article, the use of deceased donor organs for transplants that fail to meet standard donor criteria and the legitimacy of interventions and research aimed at optimizing their successful donation are discussed.

Candidates for abdominal transplant undergo a pretransplant evaluation to identify associated conditions that may require intervention or that may influence a patient's candidacy for transplant. Coronary artery disease is prevalent in candidates for abdominal organ transplantation. The optimal approach to identify and manage coronary artery disease in the peri-transplant period is currently unclear. In liver transplant candidates portopulmonary hypertension and hepatopulmonary syndrome should be screened for. Identification of the patient who is too sick to benefit from transplant is problematic; with no good evidence available decisions should be individualized and made after multidisciplinary discussion.

Patients undergoing abdominal organ transplantation have extensive comorbidities that can affect many organ systems including the cardiovascular system. Intraoperative anesthesia care can be very challenging and requires thorough understanding of the disease specific physiology as well as knowledge of the comorbidities and the surgical procedure. There is no approach to intraoperative anesthesia care that will work equally well for every center but standardization of protocols for each transplant center will improve patient care and safety and ultimately contributes to superior outcomes. In this article we provide background and suggestions that will help with the development of standardized protocols for intraoperative management.

Critical care of the general surgical patient requires synthesis of the patient's physiology, intraoperative events, and preexisting comorbidities. Evaluating an abdominal solid-organ transplant recipient after surgery adds a new dimension to clinical decisions because the transplanted allograft has undergone its own physiologic challenges and now must adapt to a new environment. This donor-recipient interaction forms the foundation for assessment of early allograft function (EAF). The intensivist must accurately assess and support EAF within the context of the recipient's current physiology and preexisting comorbidities. Optimizing EAF is essential because allograft failure is a significant predictor of recipient morbidity and mortality.

Mitchell Sally and Darren Malinoski

A shortage of organs is available for transplantation, with 116,000 patients on the Organ Procurement and Transplantation Network/United Network for Organ Sharing wait list. Because the demand for organs outweighs the supply, considerable care must be taken to maximize the number of organs transplanted per donor and optimize the quality of recovered organs. Studies designed to determine optimal donor management therapies are limited, and this research has many challenges. Although evidenced-based guidelines for managing potential organ donors do not exist, research in this area is increasing. This article reviews the existing literature and highlights recent trials that can guide management.

Zoltan Hevesi and Laura Hammel

The United States exhibits subpar health care outcomes compared with the Organisation for Economic Co-operation and Development peer group. An urgent need exists to address the excessive cost and unsustainable trajectory of expenditures associated with US health care. Health care reform ideas based on the Health Maintenance Organization and Patient-Centered Medical Home concepts are a promising solution to address health care inefficiencies. Accountable Care Organizations seek to simultaneously improve quality of care and reduce expenditure.

ANESTHESIOLOGY CLINICS

FORTHCOMING ISSUES

March 2014
Pediatric Anesthesiology
Alan Schwartz, Dean Andropolous,
and Andrew Davidson, *Editors*

June 2014
Ambulatory Anesthesia
Jeffrey Apfelbaum, and
Thomas Cutter, *Editors*

September 2014
Vascular Anesthesia
Charles Hill, *Editor*

RECENT ISSUES

September 2013
Obstetric Anesthesia
Robert Gaiser, *Editor*

June 2013
Cardiac Anesthesia
Colleen G. Koch, *Editor*

March 2013
Trauma
Yoram G. Weiss, MD, MBA, FCCM and
Micha Y. Shamir, MD, *Editors*

RELATED INTEREST

Pediatric Clinics of North America, April 2010 (Volume 57, Issue 2)
Optimization of Outcomes for Children After Solid Organ Transplantation
Vicky Lee Ng and Sandy Feng, *Editors*

Preface

Abdominal Transplantation

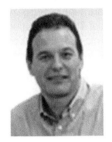

Claus U. Niemann, MD
Editor

Solid organ transplantation is now performed in hundreds of academic and private hospitals across the nation, with most of them being kidney and liver transplants. Patient outcome has dramatically improved over recent decades due to significant advances in immunosuppression and perioperative care of transplant patients. A well-defined, protocol-driven multidisciplinary team approach has been established in most transplant centers; thus transplant services are well ahead of most other surgical service lines. At a minimum, institutional protocols define preoperative, intraoperative, and postoperative management of these complex patients. Increasingly, these protocols are often built on evidence-based information rather than single institutional experience.

Organ transplantation is exceedingly complex and involves many steps well beyond matching the right organ to the right patient. An enormous logistical infrastructure is required before an organ is even offered for transplantation. In fact, considering organs as distinct biological systems in deceased donors (which by federal law are no longer human subjects) is an increasingly recognized paradigm that has led to donor management goals and a national performance metrics that closely tracks organ function and organ recovery rate.

Organ transplantation is very transparent with center-specific patient waitlists and transplant outcomes readily available online for the public. A regular comprehensive (some may argue too comprehensive) review of transplant centers, organ procurement organizations, and histocompatibility laboratories are performed by the United Network of Organ Sharing (UNOS), which is directly contracted by the Department of Health and Human Services to oversee the transplantation in the United States.

In summary, transplantation in the United States has already many elements of care delivery models that are envisioned with accountable care organizations. A highly specialized group of multidisciplinary physicians provide care to a specific patient

Anesthesiology Clin 31 (2013) ix–x
http://dx.doi.org/10.1016/j.anclin.2013.09.006
1932-2275/13/$ – see front matter © 2013 Elsevier Inc. All rights reserved.

population. The care and outcomes of these patients are constantly evaluated with a robust quality metrics that allows evaluation of overall patient care, cost, and quality.

Claus U. Niemann, MD
Department of Anesthesia and Perioperative Care
Department of Surgery
Division of Transplantation
University of California San Francisco
521 Parnassus Avenue
San Francisco, CA 94143-0648, USA

E-mail address:
Claus.Niemann@ucsf.edu

Advances in Transplantation 1940–2014

Michael Ramsay, MD, FRCA

KEYWORDS

- History • Transplantation • Liver • Kidney • Pancreas • Intestinal

KEY POINTS

- The history of medicine is that what was inconceivable yesterday and barely achievable today often becomes routine tomorrow.
- Liver transplantation began with almost no resources at the same time as the tentative first steps were taken to land a man on the moon. Because human lives would be at stake, both objectives had a sacramental element from the outset: a solemnly binding commitment to perfection.
- "I asked whether the patient could receive a kidney transplant and was told 'it can't be done'."
- The gift of an organ is really a gift of life, and something as valuable as a life-saving organ is more important to a suffering patient than wealth or power.
- The concept of a team approach to the care of the transplant patient is an important factor in the development of a successful program. This has resulted in recipient survival rates reaching 90% at one year.

INTRODUCTION

"At the present state of our knowledge, renal homotransplants do not appear to be justified in the treatment of human disease."[1–5] The 1950s and 1960s shaped the future of major organ transplantation. The major advances were associated with the understanding and development of immunosuppressive agents, and the success of techniques for organ preservation. Experimental transplantation of kidneys between animals and between animals and humans had been performed without success. Alexis Carrel described the technique of vascular anastomosis but realized that unless some method of preventing the recipient from reacting against this foreign tissue was developed, there would be no future for organ transplantation.

In working with skin grafts, Peter Medawar was able to show that failure of a graft was an immunologic response.[6] In 1953, Medawar also described acquired tolerance,

Disclosures: None.
Department of Anesthesiology and Pain Management, Baylor University Medical Center, 3500 Gaston Avenue, Dallas, TX 75246, USA
E-mail address: docram@baylorhealth.edu

Anesthesiology Clin 31 (2013) 645–658
http://dx.doi.org/10.1016/j.anclin.2013.08.001

anesthesiology.theclinics.com

offering an opportunity that organs might be accepted if the immune system was manipulated appropriately.[7] The initial strategies to combat rejection included total body irradiation and adrenal cortical steroids. These approaches had minimal effect, but the antileukemia drug 6-mercaptopurine prolonged renal allograft survival in dogs.[8] This development resulted in the discovery that azathioprine had immuno-suppression properties.[9] However, the results were not impressive, until Starzl combined it with prednisone and showed that rejection could be prevented and, if present, reversed.[10] This advance allowed the success and future of major organ transplantation.

KIDNEY TRANSPLANTATION

In 1936, Russian surgeon Yu Yu Voronoy transplanted a kidney into the groin of a patient suffering from mercury poisoning. This was an attempt to tide the patient over an acute episode of anuria. This attempt failed, but in 1945, Landsteiner and Hufnagel did transplant a kidney from a cadaver to the brachial artery and cephalic vein of a young woman in acute renal failure. The patient's own kidneys resumed function a few hours later and the transplant was excised. No details of the anesthesia are given for these procedures or any later attempts until the first successful renal transplant in 1954.[5]

On December 23, 1954, the first successful kidney transplant was performed by surgeons Joseph Murray and Hartwell Harrison, together with nephrologist John Merrill (**Fig. 1**). The donor and recipient were identical twins, 1 twin healthy and the other dying of renal disease. The operation was successful and the recipient survived for more than 2 decades. He did have to go back to surgery to have his native kidneys removed because of continuing hypertension. The donated kidney underwent 82 minutes of warm ischemia time and yet functioned promptly on reperfusion.[11]

The management of anesthesia presented much concern.[12] First, consenting the living donor to undergo a procedure that had no potential benefit to him at all was carefully evaluated. The hospital medical staff and Board of Trustees approved it and the Supreme Court of Massachusetts passed a declaratory judgment allowing the operations to proceed. The anesthetic plan for the donor was to give the most near-perfect anesthetic. This plan required the assignment of an experienced

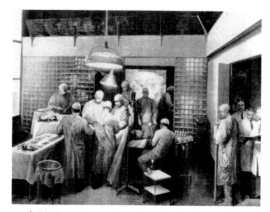

Fig. 1. The first successful kidney transplantation. Note the recipient is under spinal anesthesia. (*From* The First Successful Organ Transplantation in Man, oil on linen, 70 × 88 inches, 1996. Harvard Medical Library in the Francis A. Countway Library of Medicine. *Courtesy of* Joel Babb; with permission.)

anesthetist, and giving him rein to choose the anesthetic safest in his hands. General anesthesia was used, and in the first donor, brisk hemorrhage occurred when the entire renal artery was taken, not leaving a cuff on the aorta that could be clamped, so digital control was necessary. The anesthetic choice made was nitrous oxide, oxygen, and ether, together with tracheal intubation. The use of ether was determined to be safe in the presence of cautery if the cautery was at least 0.6 m (2 feet) away from the face and the ether was administered via a tight seal around the airway.

The recipient presented in renal failure together with hypertension, congestive heart failure, and encephalopathy. Concern for potassium intoxication required monitoring of the electrocardiogram and care with transfusion of banked blood, because this would add excess potassium. Further concerns about the recipient being particularly prone to infection called for strict reverse isolation precautions. The anesthetic equipment was sterilized, and the anesthetist was gowned and gloved. The anesthetic used for the recipient was a continuous spinal technique. This decision appeared to be logical because this was a lower abdominal extraperitoneal surgical procedure, requiring little or no muscle relaxation. The development of hypotension was not a problem with the spinal anesthetic, because these patients were hypertensive as a result of their kidney disease. Occasional small amounts of intravenous thiopental were administered if the patient became anxious. The report of the initial anesthetic technique by Vandam was followed by a conclusion that anesthesiologists would contribute to the care of transplant recipients, as part of a multidisciplinary approach, as transplants become more frequent, when the immune response is solved.

As experience with kidney transplantation increased, further reports of anesthesia management were described. In 1964, Levine and Virtue[13] described the experience of the first 50 renal transplants at the University of Colorado. These investigators noted that the surgeon required a quiet and well-relaxed patient and that the recipient required analgesia. The living donor procedures required more time than a standard nephrectomy, approximately 5 hours 45 minutes, and organ hypothermia was being used to protect the graft. The investigators also described that recipients who underwent pretransplant dialysis on the artificial kidney experienced a decrease in cholinesterase concentration, making them susceptible to prolonged paralysis if succinylcholine was administered. The investigators also raised the question of cardiac arrhythmias as a result of potassium changes if succinylcholine was administered to a patient in renal failure.

Strunin[14] reported on some aspects of anesthesia for renal homotransplantation, describing the first 36 patients receiving cadaveric (the term cadaveric is no longer in use and has been replaced by deceased donor) kidneys at St Mary's Hospital in London, United Kingdom. When cadaveric donors are used, the importance of keeping the total ischemia time short was recognized, and this placed the transplant team on 24-hour response availability.[15] The added protection of the homograft by ice-cooling was described by Calne,[16] and this proved that a more prolonged ischemia could be withstood. At the time, this period could be experimentally as much as 12 hours and this and longer times are now possible in clinical practice for some grafts. The recipients were noted to all be young in this series (11–44 years), and to have similar major clinical and biomedical disturbances. They were generally severely debilitated, anemic, hypertensive, metabolic acidotic, uremic, hyperkalemic, and hyponatremic. A general anesthetic technique was used, with intravenous thiopentone and succinylcholine in the more compensated patients or cyclopropane and oxygen in the less compensated patients. The airway was secured, mechanical ventilation instituted and hemodynamics were closely controlled. Bradycardia was noted with repeat doses of succinylcholine and was treated with atropine. The use of muscle relaxants not excreted by the kidney was recommended, and concerns about potentially lethal increases in serum potassium were raised, particularly if there was a need for transfusion of banked blood. Continuous monitoring with the electrocardiogram was recommended to detect early cardiac changes caused by increased serum potassium levels.

Increased experience with renal transplantation and anesthesia resulted in more case series being reported.[17] Katz and colleagues reported concerns with prolonged curarization in some patients if tubocurare was administered and supported the use of succinylcholine. These investigators also recommended that vasopressors should be administered only if hypotension was severe enough to cause a reduction in renal blood flow. Adequate fluid replacement was recommended.

In 1971, Powell and Golby[18] questioned the use of succinylcholine after reports[19] of fatal hyperkalemic cardiac arrest in patients with hyperkalemic renal insufficiency succinylcholine continues to be used in some centers when the patient is normokalemic.

In 1972, the University of Colorado experience in renal transplantation had increased to almost 300 cases, and Aldrete and colleagues[20] reported on their experience with 260 recipient anesthetics. These investigators concluded that most recipients were young patients with high anesthetic risk. The choice of anesthetic had to take into account how the drugs were metabolized and excreted and that renal function may not appear immediately after reperfusion of the graft. Complications noted were hypotension, cardiac arrhythmias including 2 arrests, temperature changes, and failure to detoxify anesthetic agents.

A review by Monks and Lumley[21] on anesthetic aspects of renal transplantation recommended the monitoring of central venous pressure to more accurately manage volume (**Fig. 2**).

In recent years, the improved tissue crossmatching of donors and recipients, improved immunosuppression techniques, and the availability of perfusion pumps to maintain the integrity of a graft before implantation have resulted in a success rate higher than 90% for a functioning organ more than 1 year after kidney transplantation and recipient survival at 5 years of more than 85%.[22]

LIVER TRANSPLANTATION

After the success of renal transplantation, the experiences learned were applied to liver transplantation. In the mid 1950s, the technical feasibility of orthotopic liver transplantation had been shown in dogs, but the required immunosuppression

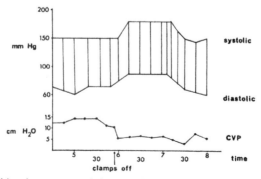

Fig. 2. Increase in blood pressure and decrease in central venous pressure after revascularization of a kidney. (*From* Monks PS, Lumley J. Anesthetic aspects of renal transplantation. Ann R Coll Surg Engl 1972;50:357; with permission.)

had not been elucidated.[23] The appreciation that azathioprine and prednisone administered together could provide immunosuppression allowed liver transplantation in humans to proceed.[10] Tom Starzl at the University of Colorado made the first 4 attempts in 1963. The anesthesia team included Antonio Aldrete and the late David LaVine. The first recipient bled to death during the operation, and the next 4 patients survived the surgery but died between 6 and 23 days later. This experience was followed by a moratorium on liver transplants at this center until 1967, when an additional immunosuppression drug became available: antilymphocyte globulin. Five of the next 25 liver transplant recipients survived for a year or more. The reasons for failure were analyzed and determined to be technical; failure because of bile duct reconstruction resulted in untreatable infections. Addressing these issues, the 1-year survival in 30 consecutive patients increased to 50%.[24] Aldrete and colleagues[25] documented the anesthesia experience in managing 25 of these patients. The preoperative condition of the recipients was described, including respiratory and cardiovascular changes. Many of the signs and symptoms of hepatopulmonary syndrome were described, as were those of cardiomyopathy. Despite the lack of conclusive evidence at the time that halothane was potentially hepatotoxic, the anesthesia team prudently elected not to use it, they used fluoroxene. The hemodynamic changes in 1 patient undergoing orthotopic liver transplantation were recorded (**Fig. 3**). The effects of major venous vessel clamping on the circulation were described, as were electrolyte and acid-base changes.

Another early report on the anesthetic management of patients undergoing liver transplantation came from Sir Roy Calne's team in Cambridge, United Kingdom.[26] These investigators reviewed the anesthetic management of the first 27 patients to receive orthotopic liver transplants at their center. A standard technique of barbiturate induction and endotracheal intubation with succinylcholine and cricoid pressure was

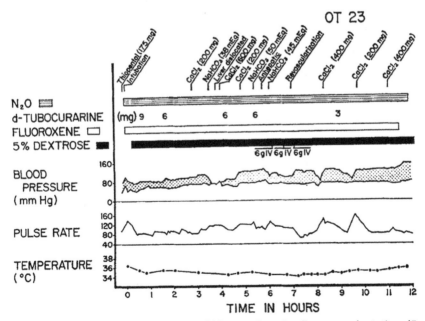

Fig. 3. Intraoperative record of a 15-year-old boy undergoing liver transplantation. (*From* Aldrete JA, LeVine DS, Gingrich TF. Experience in anesthesia for liver transplantation. Anesth Analg 1969;48:808; with permission.)

used, along with maintenance using nitrous oxide muscle relaxant and occasional low concentration of inhalational agent. Direct monitoring of arterial pressure and central venous pressure was instituted. Fresh blood was used when possible to treat blood loss and coagulopathy. Calcium chloride was administered to prevent citrate toxicity with blood transfusion. Changes in hemodynamics during the liver transplantation were summarized (**Fig. 4**). Changes in body temperature were recorded as the cold graft was reperfused into the recipient (**Fig. 5**).

A report by Farman and colleagues[26] emphasized the biochemical changes that occur during liver transplantation and included an early description of the reperfusion syndrome. These early reports of anesthetic management of liver transplantation reflected the problems encountered during this procedure.

The major advance in liver transplantation was the development of an effective immunosuppressant drug, cyclosporine. Calne and his team were able to show both experimentally and clinically the effectiveness of cyclosporine.[27,28] This discovery allowed the critically ill liver recipient who could not tolerate the required doses of azathioprine and steroids to undergo the rigors of transplantation and survive. The survival rates of liver recipients increased from 25% to more than 75%, and thus cyclosporine became the backbone of successful liver transplantation.[29] The immunologic and technical challenges of removing a diseased liver in a debilitated patient with portal hypertension, coagulopathy, electrolyte derangements, and major organ dysfunction and implanting a new graft that has sustained ischemia required a specialized team of experts in all fields of medicine. A dedicated group of anesthesiologists allowed many of these major perioperative derangements to be addressed and best practices to be developed and disseminated through publications, meetings, and word of mouth.[30] Many centers published reports of the early perioperative management of liver transplantation and identified the major problems, which needed more research and resources to be tackled successfully.

In 1981, Starzl had moved his team to the University of Pittsburgh, which became a major resource for physicians from around the world to visit, learn, and contribute to transplantation. Symposia were held and a multidisciplinary society was formed, named the International Society for Perioperative Care in Liver Transplantation. This society later became known as the International Liver Transplantation Society, with

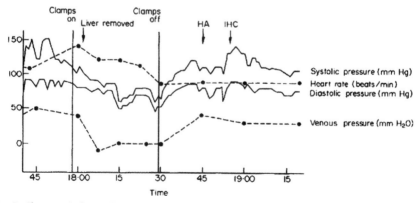

Fig. 4. Changes in hemodynamics during liver transplantation. Vertical lines indicate anhepatic period. HA, hepatic artery anastomosis complete; IHC, infrahepatic cava anastomosis complete. (*From* Farman JV, Lines JG, Williams RS, et al. Liver transplantation in man. Anesthetic and biochemical management. Anesthesia 1974;29:22; with permission.)

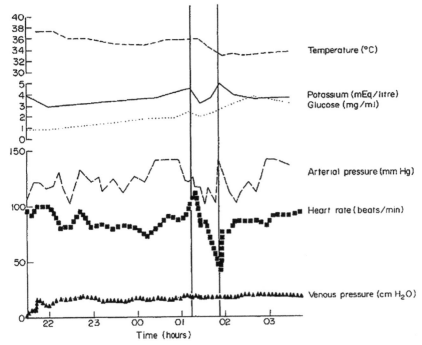

Fig. 5. Changes in temperature, potassium, glucose, and hemodynamics during liver transplantation. (*From* Farman JV, Lines JG, Williams RS, et al. Liver transplantation in man. Anesthetic and biochemical management. Anesthesia 1974;29:26; with permission.)

a mission to emphasize the multidisciplinary approach to liver transplantation and provide a forum for communication between clinicians, scientists, and researchers from all disciplines with an interest in transplantation. In addition to meetings, a peer-reviewed journal, and worldwide representation, the society has developed a Web site, which makes the latest publications, lectures, and videos on liver transplantation immediately available to its membership.[31]

COAGULOPATHY

The liver has a major function in balancing the coagulation system. Severe derangements in coagulation may occur as a result of liver cirrhosis and also as a result of undergoing a liver transplant and reperfusion of the new graft. Major bleeding may also occur as a result of portal hypertension and large varices. The need to be able to transfuse large volumes of blood rapidly resulted in the design of a rapid infusion device. These devices have become routine in the management of major trauma surgery (**Fig. 6**).

Routine laboratory tests do not give a real-time picture of the state of coagulation. The University of Pittsburgh team introduced the thrombelastograph, a whole blood, real-time assessment of global coagulation and fibrinolysis during liver transplantation (**Fig. 7**).[32]

The value of technologies like thrombelastography was confirmed by Armando Tripodi, who showed that the coagulopathy of liver cirrhosis was a balance between the procoagulant and anticoagulant factors produced by the liver.[33] A hypercoaguable

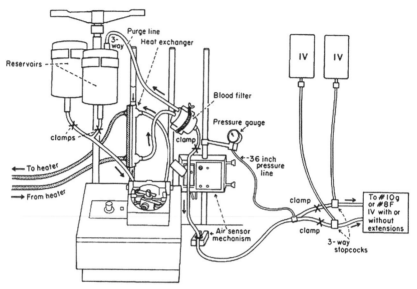

Fig. 6. A rapid infusion system developed at the University of Pittsburgh. (*From* Kang YG, Martin DJ, Marquez J, et al. Intraoperative changes in blood coagulation and thrombelasto-graphic monitoring in liver transplantation. Anesth Analg 1985;64:889; with permission.)

state could exist despite a prothrombin time of 18 seconds. This situation is because the liver also synthesizes anticoagulant factors such as protein C, protein S, and antithrombin. The resulting imbalance may result in a hypercoagulant state, which may be easily detected by thrombelastography but not by routine laboratory tests.

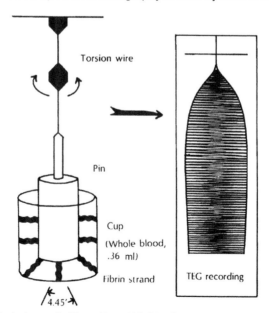

Fig. 7. The thrombelastograph. (*From* Kang YG, Martin DJ, Marquez J, et al. Intraoperative changes in blood coagulation and thrombelastographic monitoring in liver transplantation. Anesth Analg 1985;64:890; with permission.)

Cardiovascular System

The presence of a hyperkinetic circulation in the patient with liver cirrhosis has been observed for many years. This observation has made the cardiac function look good as the heart beats against a very low vascular resistance; however, in certain patients, a cardiomyopathy has been noticed, which is believed to be the result of alcoholic damage to the heart muscle. However, studies in the 1990s showed that cardiomyopathy in the form of impaired ventricular contractile responsiveness can be identified in nearly all patients with cirrhosis.[34] Clinical features of the progression of cirrhotic cardiomyopathy are represented in **Fig. 8.**

This and other pulmonary vascular disorders found in cirrhotic patients with portal hypertension such as portopulmonary hypertension and hepatopulmonary syndrome have caused clinicians, including anesthesiologists, critical care physicians, and other specialists, to study these conditions. The impact of these conditions on the outcome of liver transplantation has led to management protocols being put in place and new therapies and management techniques being developed.[35] The importance of right ventricular function has been recognized, because dysfunction of this ventricle causes graft distension and failure.[36,37] This situation has resulted in the frequent use of transesophageal echocardiographic (TEE) and transthoracic echocardiographic assessment perioperatively of liver transplant recipients.[38] The use of TEE by the liver transplant anesthesiologist is common and is best suited to detect ventricular dysfunction, left ventricular outflow obstruction, increased right ventricular systolic pressure, and the need to assess pulmonary artery hemodynamics.[39] Intracardiac thromboemboli have been observed during liver transplantation with TEE monitoring usually after reperfusion (**Fig. 9**).[40,41]

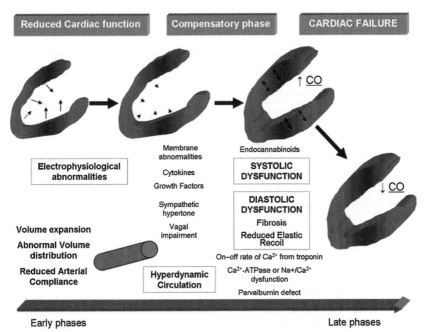

Fig. 8. The clinical features of the progression of cirrhotic cardiomyopathy. (*From* Zardi EM, Abbate A, Zardi DM, et al. Cirrhotic cardiomyopathy. J Am Coll Cardiol 2010;56:540; with permission.)

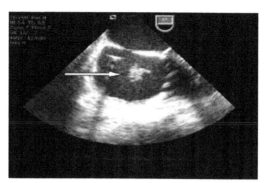

Fig. 9. TEE showing intracardiac thrombus. *Arrow* points to intraventricular embolus. (*From* Xia VW, Ho JK, Nourmand H, et al. Incidental intracardiac thromboemboli during liver transplantation: incidence, risk factors, and management. Liver Transpl 2010;16:1423; with permission.)

To improve venous return during the anhepatic phase of liver transplantation, some centers have used a venous bypass system without systemic anticoagulation.[42,43] Venous blood is drained from the portal and femoral veins and returned to the axillary vein via a centrifugal pump. Later, the return blood is passed through a percutaneously placed cannula in the internal jugular vein. However, the data on the benefit of venous bypass have not been conclusively verified, and therefore, this procedure is not used in many centers.[44,45]

These advances in liver transplantation involved anesthesiologists as an integral part of the team to varying degrees. The American Society of Anesthesiologists (http://www.asa.org/) and the United Network for Organ Sharing (http://www.unos.org/) have produced the specific requirements for providing anesthesia services for liver transplant procedures (see article by Kandula and colleagues elsewhere in this issue on allocation of resources and federal regulations for organ transplantation).

Pancreas and Islet Transplantation

Improved immunosuppression has also allowed better outcomes with pancreas transplantation. However, these grafts still face higher postoperative complications than liver or kidney grafts. This situation may be the result of rejection, graft thrombosis, or infection. Frequently, the pancreas is transplanted with a kidney because the patient has diabetic renal failure.[46] The University of Pittsburgh reported reduced rejection and thrombosis rates using a preconditioning protocol with tacrolimus. These investigators also carried out some technical refinements.[47]

Pancreatic islets cells are transplanted in a few centers that have the capability to separate the islets cells and have been reinfused into the portal vein, resulting in some diabetic recipients becoming insulin free. The success depends heavily on the islet cell load that can be prepared for reinfusion.[48]

Intestinal Transplantation

The only alternative form of treatment of patients with short gut syndrome who are dependent on total parenteral nutrition is an intestinal transplant. The early attempts at intestinal transplantation had poor success because of the lack of effective immunosuppression despite the use of cyclosporine. The inclusion of the liver with the small intestine was more successful in preventing rejection.[49] The development of a new immunosuppression drug, FK 506, was found to be more effective at protecting intestinal transplants, and they became more successful.[50] The results from the first 45 intestinal transplants performed at the University of Pittsburgh under FK 506 immunosuppression showed a 1-year patient survival of 82% and graft survival of 73%.[51]

The Future of Transplantation

There is a shortage of available organs for patients on the waiting list, and the gap between supply and demand continues to grow. This situation means that the donor pool needs to be expanded, which entails increasing the use of marginal grafts, and in the Western world, increasing the number of living donors, especially for kidney transplantation. The use of living donors exposes a healthy patient to a degree of morbidity and possible mortality. Living donor kidney transplants performed laparoscopically are becoming more routine. This procedure can allow a recipient to receive a kidney before undergoing dialysis, with its well-known complications. The cold ischemia time is also usually minimal; therefore, an excellent functioning organ can be expected. Living liver donors are at greater risk of morbidity and mortality than kidney donors. Good perfusion of the liver is required while the organ is dissected and either the right or left lobe is used as the graft. To reduce blood loss, many centers keep the central venous pressure low, to reduce the size of the liver venous reservoir. Most centers use the left lobe of the liver as there are fewer complications than with the right lobe.

Organs that are taken using extended donor criteria, such as non-heart–beating donors, elderly donors, or those with significant steatosis, are more prone to preservation-induced injury. Hypothermic machine perfusion of kidney grafts has been shown to significantly reduce the risk of delayed graft function and improve graft function in the first year after transplantation.[22] This advantage may provide better outcomes for extended criteria donor organs. This development has renewed research and interest into machine perfusion for liver grafts.[52] Various techniques have been researched: hypothermic, normothermic, and subnormothermic. It is likely that some form of machine perfusion will enter clinical liver transplantation in the near future.[53]

REFERENCES

1. Starzl TE, Iwatsuki S, Van Thiel DH, et al. Evolution of liver transplantation. Hepatology 1982;2:614–36.
2. Starzl TE, Fung JJ. Themes of liver transplantation. Hepatology 2010;51:1869–84.
3. Calne RY. It can't be done. Nat Med 2012;18:1493–5.
4. Ramsay MA. Anesthesia for liver transplantation. In: Busuttil, Klintmalm, editors. Transplantation of the liver. 2nd edition. Philadelphia: Elsevier Saunders; 2005. p. 590.
5. Hume DM, Merrill JP, Miller BF, et al. Experiences with renal homotransplantation in the human: report of nine cases. J Clin Invest 1955;34:327–82.
6. Starzl TE. Peter Brian Medawar: father of transplantation. J Am Coll Surg 1995;180:332–6.
7. Billingham RE, Brent L, Medawar PB. Actively acquired tolerance of foreign cells. Nature 1953;172:603–6.

8. Calne RY. The rejection of renal homografts. Inhibition in dogs by 6-mercaptopurine. Lancet 1960;1:417–8.

9. Calne RY. Inhibition of the rejection of renal homografts in dogs by purine analogues. Transplant Bull 1961;28:65–81.

10. Starzl TE, Marchioro TL, Waddell WR. The reversal of rejection in human renal homografts with subsequent development of homograft tolerance. Surg Gynecol Obstet 1963;117:385–95.

11. Starzl TE. The development of clinical renal transplantation. Am J Kidney Dis 1990;16:548–56.

12. Vandam LD, Harrison JH, Murray JE, et al. Anesthetic aspects of renal homotransplantation in man. With notes on the anesthetic care of the uremic patient. Anesthesiology 1962;23:783–92.

13. LeVine DS, Virtue RW. Anaesthetic agents and techniques for renal homotransplants. Can Anaesth Soc J 1964;11:425–8.

14. Strunin L. Some aspects of anaesthesia for renal homotransplantation. Br J Anaesth 1966;38:812–22.

15. Calne RY, Loughridge LW, Pryse-Davies J, et al. Renal transplantation in man: a report of five cases, using cadaveric donors. Br Med J 1963;2:645–51.

16. Calne RY, Pegg DE, Pryse-Davies J, et al. Renal preservation by ice-cooling: an experimental study relating to kidney transplantation from cadavers. Br Med J 1963;2:651–5.

17. Katz J, Kountz SL, Cohn R. Anesthetic considerations for renal transplant. Anesth Analg 1967;46:609–13.

18. Powell JN, Golby M. The pattern of potassium liberation following a single dose of suxamethonium in normal and uraemic rats. Br J Anaesth 1971;43:662–8.

19. Roth F, Wuthrich H. The clinical importance of hyperkalaemia following suxamethonium administration. Br J Anaesth 1969;41:311–6.

20. Aldrete JA, Daniel W, O'Higgins JW, et al. Analysis of anesthetic-related morbidity in human recipients of renal homografts. Anesth Analg 1971;50:321–9.

21. Monks PS, Lumley J. Anaesthetic aspects of renal transplantation. Ann R Coll Surg Engl 1972;50:354–66.

22. Moers C, Smits JM, Maathuis MH, et al. Machine perfusion or cold storage in deceased-donor kidney transplantation. N Engl J Med 2009;360:7–19.

23. Starzl TE. The succession from kidney to liver transplantation. Transplant Proc 1981;13:50–4.

24. Starzl TE, Koep LJ, Halgrimson CG, et al. Fifteen years of clinical liver transplantation. Gastroenterology 1979;77:375–88.

25. Aldrete JA, LeVine DS, Gingrich TF. Experience in anesthesia for liver transplantation. Anesth Analg 1969;48:802–14.

26. Farman JV, Lines JG, Williams RS, et al. Liver transplantation in man. Anaesthetic and biochemical management. Anaesthesia 1974;29:17–32.

27. Calne RY, White DJ, Rolles K, et al. Prolonged survival of pig orthotopic heart grafts treated with cyclosporin A. Lancet 1978;1:1183–5.

28. Calne RY, White DJ, Thiru S, et al. Cyclosporin A in patients receiving renal allografts from cadaver donors. Lancet 1978;2:1323–7.

29. Starzl TE, Klintmalm GB, Porter KA, et al. Liver transplantation with use of cyclosporin a and prednisone. N Engl J Med 1981;305:266–9.

30. Wall WJ. Liver transplantation: past accomplishments and future challenges. Can J Gastroenterol 1999;13:257–63.

31. Available at: http://iltseducation.org. Accessed September 9, 2013.
32. Kang YG, Martin DJ, Marquez J, et al. Intraoperative changes in blood coagulation and thrombelastographic monitoring in liver transplantation. Anesth Analg 1985;64:888–96.
33. Caldwell SH, Hoffman M, Lisman T, et al. Coagulation disorders and hemostasis in liver disease: pathophysiology and critical assessment of current management. Hepatology 2006;44:1039–46.
34. Ma Z, Lee SS. Cirrhotic cardiomyopathy: getting to the heart of the matter. Hepatology 1996;24:451–9.
35. Rodriguez-Roisin R, Krowka MJ, Herve P, et al. Pulmonary-hepatic vascular disorders (PHD). Eur Respir J 2004;24:861–80.
36. Ramsay M. Portopulmonary hypertension and right heart failure in patients with cirrhosis. Curr Opin Anaesthesiol 2010;23:145–50.
37. Rosendal C, Almamat Uulu K, De Simone R, et al. Right ventricular function during orthotopic liver transplantation: three-dimensional transesophageal echocardiography and thermodilution. Ann Transplant 2012;17:21–30.
38. Raval Z, Harinstein ME, Skaro AI, et al. Cardiovascular risk assessment of the liver transplant candidate. J Am Coll Cardiol 2011;58:223–31.
39. Hage FG, Bravo PE, Zoghbi GJ, et al. Hypertrophic obstructive cardiomyopathy in liver transplant patients. Cardiol J 2008;15:74–9.
40. Xia VW, Ho JK, Nourmand H, et al. Incidental intracardiac thromboemboli during liver transplantation: incidence, risk factors, and management. Liver Transpl 2010;16:1421–7.
41. Ellis JE, Lichtor JL, Feinstein SB, et al. Right heart dysfunction, pulmonary embolism, and paradoxical embolization during liver transplantation. A transesophageal two-dimensional echocardiographic study. Anesth Analg 1989;68:777–82.
42. Denmark SW, Shaw BW Jr, Starzl TE, et al. Veno-venous bypass without systemic anticoagulation in canine and human liver transplantation. Surg Forum 1983;34:380–2.
43. Shaw BW Jr, Martin DJ, Marquez JM, et al. Venous bypass in clinical liver transplantation. Ann Surg 1984;200:524–34.
44. Gurusamy KS, Koti R, Pamecha V, et al. Veno-venous bypass versus none for liver transplantation. Cochrane Database Syst Rev 2011;(3):CD007712.
45. Walia A, Mandell MS, Mercaldo N, et al. Anesthesia for liver transplantation in US academic centers: institutional structure and perioperative care. Liver Transpl 2012;18:737–43.
46. Sutherland DE, Gruessner RW, Dunn DL, et al. Lessons learned from more than 1,000 pancreas transplants at a single institution. Ann Surg 2001;233:463–501.
47. Thai NL, Abu-Elmagd K, Khan A, et al. Pancreatic transplantation at the University of Pittsburgh. Clin Transpl 2004;18:205–14.
48. Takita M, Matsumoto S, Noguchi H, et al. One hundred human pancreatic islet isolations at Baylor Research Institute. Proc (Bayl Univ Med Cent) 2010;23:341–8.
49. Grant D, Wall W, Mimeault R, et al. Successful small-bowel/liver transplantation. Lancet 1990;335:181–4.
50. Tzakis AG, Todo S, Reyes J, et al. Intestinal transplantation in children under FK 506 immunosuppression. J Pediatr Surg 1993;28:1040–3.
51. Tzakis AG, Todo S, Starzl TE. Intestinal transplantation. Annu Rev Med 1994;45:79–91.

52. Guarrera JV, Henry SD, Samstein B, et al. Hypothermic machine preservation in human liver transplantation: the first clinical series. Am J Transplant 2010;10: 372–81.
53. Monbaliu D, Brassil J. Machine perfusion of the liver: past, present and future. Curr Opin Organ Transplant 2010;15:160–6.

Infrastructure, Logistics and Regulation of Transplantation
UNOS

Julie K. Heimbach, MD

KEYWORDS

- Transplantation • Organ allocation • Compliance

KEY POINTS

- Organ transplantation requires extensive coordination of complex care to be successful.
- Federal oversight of transplantation mandates the achievement of rigorous performance and compliance metrics to remain active in transplantation.

INTRODUCTION

Organ Transplantation has evolved into the standard of care for patients with end-stage organ failure. Despite considering increasingly complex transplant recipients for organs recovered from donors with increasing comorbid conditions, 1-year patient survival following kidney transplantation is 97% in the United States, whereas liver transplant recipient 1-year survival is 90%.[1] There were 16,485 kidney recipients in the United States in 2012 and 6256 patients who underwent liver transplantation. Including recipients of thoracic organs as well as other abdominal transplantations, including pancreas and small intestine, there were 28,051 transplants performed last year.[2] With outcomes and volumes at such a high level, transplantation may seem at first glance to have become a rather routine procedure; however, when considering the number of steps that must be perfectly orchestrated to have a successful outcome, it remains quite a unique and remarkable accomplishment. The intent of this review is to highlight the logistics required for transplantation as well as review the current oversight of transplantation.

LOGISTICS

In order for a patient with organ failure to receive a transplant, they must be evaluated, accepted, and placed on the transplant waiting list by a designated transplant program. A transplant program may be part of a larger transplant center that includes

Division of Transplantation Surgery, Mayo Clinic, 200 First Street SW, Rochester, MN 55905, USA
E-mail address: heimbach.julie@mayo.edu

Anesthesiology Clin 31 (2013) 659–666
http://dx.doi.org/10.1016/j.anclin.2013.08.003
1932-2275/13/$ – see front matter © 2013 Elsevier Inc. All rights reserved.

multiple programs, such as liver, pancreas, heart, or lung, or may be a free-standing program within a hospital that only performs kidney transplantation. Regardless of the number of other programs within an institution, there are key components that must be in place that are both required by federal oversight to be a designated transplant program and are generally accepted to be part of best practice (**Box 1**).[3,4]

Once a patient has been accepted for transplantation, they may proceed to transplant with a living donor if living donation is possible (commonly done for kidney transplant recipients; less commonly done for liver transplant recipients; rarely done for lung transplant recipients) or they may wait for a deceased donor organ. Living donors are evaluated by transplant programs, which typically perform the donor nephrectomy or hepatectomy if the donor is approved and care for the donor following the donor surgery. As mentioned in the article by Kandula and colleagues elsewhere in this issue, deceased donors are evaluated and managed Organ Procurement Organizations (OPOs), which are organizations staffed by dedicated professionals who have many responsibilities including working with families to discuss options and obtain consent for donation, manage the care of potential donors from consent until donation occurs, and coordinating organ recovery within a geographically defined area called the Donor Service Area (DSA). DSAs are variable in both size and population served, generally arising from historical boundaries in place before federal oversight of transplantation. Primarily for the purpose of organ allocation, DSAs are further organized into 11 larger geographic areas called regions (see table 3 from the article by Kandula and colleagues elsewhere in this issue).

The responsibilities of the OPOs are extensive, including, among many things, the need to obtain consent for donation, the appropriate workup and screening for potentially transmissible donor-derived diseases, ABO verification, optimizing medical management of the donor from the time of consent to organ recovery, placement of the organs to the appropriate wait-listed candidate according to allocation policy,

---

Box 1
Transplant program requirements

1. Compliance with policies and obligations of OPTN membership and maintenance of designated transplant program status (see OPTN bylaws, Ref.[3])

2. Compliance with updated Medicare COP, for Medicare participating transplant programs only (see Ref.[4])

3. Affiliation with an approved OPO

4. Affiliation with an OPTN approved HLA laboratory

5. Sufficient blood bank support

6. Capacity to monitor immunosuppressant levels and perform microbiology and complex blood chemistry testing

7. Transplant program key personnel who meet designated criteria, including primary physician, surgeon, director of liver transplant anesthesia (if applicable), clinical transplant coordinator, transplant pharmacist, transplant mental/social support professionals, independent donor advocate and living donor surgeons (living donor programs only), nutritional support personnel (CMS only)

8. Develop and maintain protocols for the care of recipients and living donors

9. Develop and maintain active Quality Assessment and Performance Improvement programs (CMS only)

Abbreviation: COP, Certificate of Participation.

coordinating the transportation of organ recovery teams and organs, and the appropriate packaging and labeling of organs. Deceased donor abdominal organ recoveries are most commonly performed by the transplant program, which has been allocated the liver, while thoracic organs are frequently recovered by teams from the individual heart and/or lung programs. At times, a local transplant center located near the donor hospital or staff working for the OPO may perform the recovery and the organs are then transported to the recipients' transplant program. In most cases, the organ recovery occurs at the facility where the donor is hospitalized, although at times the donor may be transported to a different location for the organ recovery.

Once the recipient has been listed, and a suitable living donor is identified or a suitable deceased donor organ is allocated, and compatibility is ensured by appropriate ABO/anti-Human Leukocyte Antigen (HLA) testing, the transplant is performed. (For more details see the article by Kandula and colleagues elsewhere in this issue.) In many cases, the timing of the transplant cannot be predicted or controlled and thus transplant programs need to maintain an appropriate staffing level to be able to accommodate surgeries being performed at highly variable times with frequent clustering of cases. The condition of wait-listed candidates must be closely monitored to ensure that when an organ becomes available, the potential recipient is in a suitable condition to undergo a surgical procedure. The frequency of the follow-up is determined the patient's condition, the local medical resources available to the patient, and the ability of the local information to be communicated to the transplant center. The intraoperative complexity of liver transplantation has warranted the development of specific criteria to determine qualified anesthesia support (see section titled oversight of transplantation). In addition, specific experience and training criteria have been established for a transplant program's designated primary medical and surgical director of a transplant program. Although there is oversight of the credentials and experience of the individuals identified to serve in key roles such as primary physician or surgeon, the credentialing of supporting staff members within programs is left to the individual hospitals and medical practices.

Although living donor transplantation can be planned and scheduled, which allows for the medical condition of the recipient to be optimized, the logistics can still be challenging for centers with the need to coordinate staffing for both a donor and a recipient operating room. These logistics become even more challenging in the case of paired donation, or donor chains in which donor organs from noncompatible donor-recipient pairs are exchanged into compatible recipients, which at times may be at different hospitals, potentially even in locations many states away. Optimal timing of the recipient operation relative to the donor operation remains essential to ensure the best outcome possible.

Unlike living donor transplantation, timing of deceased donor organ transplantation is not as predictable. Although a candidate's position on the wait list relative to others can be monitored, organ donor availability is highly variable. Organ allocation policy varies depending on the type of transplant. Factors that may influence organ allocation include the medical condition of the recipient (for thoracic organs and livers), HLA matching (pancreas and kidney), pediatric versus adult, and location of the donor relative to the recipient. As mentioned in the article by Kandula and colleagues elsewhere in this issue, donor organs are typically first offered to recipients who are listed at transplant centers within the same DSA as the donor hospital, although there are many exceptions to this and this may be subject to further change in the future to reduce geographic disparity in organ availability. If an organ is accepted for a wait-listed patient within the local DSA, it may be offered wait-listed candidates within the region and then to candidates wait-listed in all regions across the United States.

Once a donor organ has been accepted for a potential recipient, the recipient must be admitted to the hospital and prepared for surgery. Centers must ensure that no new medical or social issues have arisen since the potential recipient was last evaluated or if the recipient is currently hospitalized (increasingly common for liver recipients), that their condition is stable enough to undergo transplantation at the time the organ is available. Concurrent with the recipient's arrival to the hospital, the organ recovery team(s) is typically traveling to the donor hospital to perform the organ recovery. The organ recovery is typically performed in the operating room of the donor hospital. If the donor is unstable, this may require disrupting the elective schedule, although often organ recovery occurs late in the day or in the middle of the night, which is less disruptive to the donor hospital but requires the recipient team to mobilize at odd hours. Once the organs have been cooled and flushed with preservation solution (a time typically designated as cross-clamp), due to limits of organ viability, transplantation must now occur in a timely fashion following cross-clamp. Thoracic organs are most sensitive to ischemic injury, and thus the recipient operation is frequently started before cross-clamp. The goal for implantation for livers is generally under 8 to 12 hours, although depending on the quality of the donor organ, this timing may be adjusted. For organs recovered from older donors, or from non-heart-beating donors called donation after cardiac death donors, it may be particularly beneficial to shorten the ischemic time. Pancreas and kidneys may be safely transplanted with longer ischemic times relative to liver, especially if the kidney is placed on machine perfusion pump, although as for other types of transplants, the quality of the donor organ also plays a role. In all cases, ischemic times should be minimized. Because the timing of the donor offer is not under the control of the transplant program, centers must be prepared to perform transplants at all hours of the day or night, regardless of weekend or holiday schedules. In many cases, organ offers may overlap, and centers must be able to accommodate simultaneous or sequential transplants given that it is not known when the next offer may occur.

After the transplant is performed, recipients (and living donors) typically obtain their follow-up care at the transplant center, although the length and intensity of follow-up are variable. Some centers provide follow-up for all aspects of the recipient's care for the life of recipient, whereas others manage only immunosuppression. Most centers provide care that is somewhere between these 2 levels. The publically reported outcomes for 1- and 3-year survival achieved by each center, which are closely tracked by federal oversight agencies and payers, provide strong incentive for post-transplant care.[1] In addition, programs have frequently established long-term relationships with their patients, whom they may have cared for while they were waiting for transplantation. There are, however, logistical and economic challenges to providing long-term care for recipients and donors who may not live in close proximity to the transplant center. Future innovations, such as use of social media for communication, on-line access of the electronic medical record, or video conferencing, may improve this, although an additional burden is that much of the care currently provided remotely, such as the monitoring of immunosuppression levels and adjusting of medications, is not typically part of standard coverage plans.

OVERSIGHT OF TRANSPLANTATION

Transplantation is unique in medicine in that although there is a highly effective treatment for an otherwise lethal condition (end-stage organ failure), access to that treatment remains severely limited by the extreme shortage of organs suitable for transplantation. Currently, more than 118,500 people are on the wait list, with more than 96,000 waiting for kidney transplantation and nearly 16,000 waiting for liver transplantation.[2] The availability of organs rests solely on the altruism of individuals and families who provide the life-saving gift of organ donation. Oversight is intended to ensure organs are well used, and that policies and procedures that are in place to provide as fair and equitable distribution of organs as possible are followed, which ultimately may influence public trust in the system.

As mentioned in the article by Kandula and colleagues elsewhere in this issue, The Organ Procurement and Transplantation Network (OPTN) was mandated by the National Organ Transplantation Act (NOTA) of 1984 and then further clarified in the Final Rule. NOTA requires that the OPTN be run by contract from a private entity, and this contract is currently held by United Network for Organ Sharing (UNOS). NOTA and the final rule outline specific responsibilities of the OPTN, which are as follows[5,6]:

1. Development and monitoring of compliance with policies for safe and efficient recovery of organs from transplantation
2. Establishment of equitable allocation of organs based on medical judgment
3. Establishment of training and experience requirements for key medical and surgical personnel as well as other required resources for non-Medicare transplant programs
4. Collection of data related to the performance of transplantation
5. Conduction of program reviews on behalf of the Secretary of Heath
6. Protection of the health and safety of the public as it relates to transplantation

UNOS is responsible for oversight of its members including transplant hospitals and OPOs, although it does not have regulatory authority over individual transplant providers. UNOS monitors performance metrics for transplant programs and more recently for OPOs, as well as monitoring compliance with OPTN policy through routine required data submission for all transplant activity, including donor and recipient data. In addition, UNOS generally performs routine site visits every 3 years for multiorgan transplant programs to ensure accuracy and compliance with mandatory data submission, in addition to offering peer review and due process for centers found to have policy violations.

To formulate and monitor policy, UNOS has selected members of the transplant community, including surgeons, physicians, nurses, transplant OPO personnel, and patient representatives, to voluntarily serve on national committees that are dedicated to the optimization and oversight of transplantation. There are representatives from each of the 11 regions as well as selected at-large members to ensure a broad range of perspectives on each committee. There are organ-specific committees, such as the Kidney, Liver-Intestine, and Pancreas committees, that are primarily tasked with developing policies to improve aspects of transplantation, such as optimizing organ allocation, while the Membership and Professional Standards Committee (MPSC) is tasked with the oversight of OPTN members. The 3 main areas of focus for the MPSC are reviewing applications for new programs or key personnel changes to ensure the required standards are met, monitoring of transplant center and OPO activity and outcome, and investigating potential noncompliance with OPTN policy.[7]

As previously noted, UNOS/OPTN does have specific criteria for primary surgeon and physician for each respective transplant program that specifies the training and case volume requirements needed for certification.[3] In addition, due to the unique and complex intraoperative issues of liver transplantation, liver transplant programs must also designate a Director of Liver Transplant Anesthesia, who is required to have board certification by the American Board of Anesthesia or the foreign equivalent, and to have either the completion of a critical care or liver transplant anesthesia fellowship with perioperative care of at least 10 liver transplant recipients or experience in the perioperative care within the operating room of at least 20 liver transplant recipients within the last 5 years. The Liver Transplant Anesthesia Director should also maintain at least 8 hours of continuing medical education within transplantation within the last 3 years.[3]

According to OPTN policy, transplant programs are required to achieve minimum expected outcomes. Programs with observed graft failures or patient deaths exceeding 1.5 of the risk-adjusted expected results (O/E [Observed to Expected] >1.5), provided that result is statistically significant based on a one-sided P value <.05 and that the observed number of graft failures or deaths minus the expected number is greater than 3, will be identified as not meeting the required outcome standards; this is publically available information. As previously noted, transplant programs are required by policy to submit certain mandatory data elements, including outcome data. This data are then analyzed by the Scientific Registry of Transplant Recipients, who then generate a program-specific report that encompasses data from a 2.5-year cycle with an month lag time to ensure at least 1 year of follow-up. Centers that do not meet these minimum outcome standards or are noncompliant with other aspects of OPTN policy are subject to peer review by the MPSC, which may include additional monitoring and reporting requirements, a site visit, and/or potential adverse actions. The potential adverse actions range from a letter of uncontested violation up to probation or member not in good standing. Centers may also be recommended for termination, although this action must be carried out by the Secretary of Health and Human Services.[7]

Additional oversight of transplant programs is provided by the Centers for Medicare Services (CMS) for all centers that are certified by Medicare. Historically, CMS has been involved in oversight of transplant programs, although approval was based largely on meeting certain volume and outcome data. Nonrenal transplant programs that wished to obtain Medicare certification submitted applications that were reviewed by expert panels, whereas renal programs were subjected to an on-site visit. After several widely publicized events highlighted potential gaps in transplant program oversight,[8] CMS developed a renewed oversight policy with vigorous enforcement and potential for termination of Medicare services not only for the program failing to achieve expected process and performance metrics but for all transplant programs within that center. The updated policy, adopted June 28, 2007, is termed the Certificate of Participation and overlaps with many of oversight functions of UNOS/OPTN.[4] Most importantly, CMS adopted the same flagging criteria to identify programs that are not meeting the expected graft and patient survival outcomes. There are other areas where the policy requirements are not identical or not addressed, such as the CMS requirement for written policies regarding documentation of the informed consent process and documentation of a process for quality assessment and performance improvement, neither of which are required by OPTN. This dual oversight is a challenge for centers, especially given that both CMS and UNOS conduct on-site reviews every 3 years, which last up to 1 week and require significant staff to support. CMS is considering a proposal, currently available for public comment, of whether to continue to repeat on-site visits for all programs every 3 years versus site visit only if indicated by performance metrics.

The need to achieve minimum outcome standards places significant pressure on programs to minimize risks in selection of both donors and recipients. For example, the current expected 1-year patient survival for living donor kidney recipients in the United States is 98.6%. If a transplant program performs 100 living donor kidney transplants for recipients who are of average risk, they would only be able to have approximately 3 deaths over the subsequent 12 months following transplantation to remain within the expected range. Although the data are risk adjusted, the consequences of performing below the expected level may be "sudden, severe, and soon" according to Hamilton[9] in a recent review of CMS oversight, and thus centers may feel compelled to avoid candidates whom they perceive not to be adequately risk adjusted. Similarly, despite the tremendous organ shortage, centers may avoid selecting grafts that have a higher risk of failure to decrease the potential for graft loss. Indeed, a recent survey of transplant program that was performed after the CMS oversight went into place identified that 58% had increased recipient selection criteria and 52% had increased donor selection criteria in the last 3 years.[10] Transplantation of extended criteria donor kidneys declined nationally by 13.7% from 1826 to 1617 from 2007 to 2010, and the number of extended criteria donor organs recovered across all organ types also declined during that same period by 9.3% (from 3249 to 2945).[9] An additional concern is that because expected survival is determined by actual survival for a given population, as centers make additional adjustments to their programs and achieve better outcomes (similar to a group of students studying for a test graded on a curve), the survival curve may shift inexorably toward higher and higher expected survival. This concern for the needs of the patient versus the needs of the transplant program is balanced by the potential benefits of increased oversight, which may include the adoption of standardized "best practices" and other performance improvements, which could lead to better outcomes.

Both OPTN/UNOS and CMS offer paths forward for programs not meeting the standard outcome criteria, or for other policy violations. For OPTN/UNOS, centers undergo peer review by the MPSC, which may include a site visit to identify strengths and weaknesses of the program. Centers will be offered the opportunity to improve and, if this improvement is not demonstrated, they may be considered for adverse action as previously outlined.[7] For CMS, centers not meeting criteria will be cited, although they will not be considered for termination unless they have not met criteria for 2 of the last 5 data reporting cycles including the current cycle.[4] Centers that are cited for outcomes are able to request consideration of mitigating factors, which will be ruled on after a period of 210 days. The request may be accepted outright and the center released form review, or centers may be offered the chance to enter into a "Systems Improvement Agreement," which essentially is a contract that specifies the required elements and timeline for improvement. A third scenario is that the request for mitigating factors may be denied, resulting in termination of Medicare services. Regardless of the eventual outcome of either OPTN or CMS action, the ability of centers to maintain or obtain insurance contracts may also be affected by program performance statistically below the expected level for a reporting period.

SUMMARY

Transplantation is the standard of care for selected patients with end-stage organ failure and provides the opportunity for excellent long-term survival. It does require extraordinary coordination of care before, during, and after transplantation to maximize the likelihood of success. Transplantation depends on the availability of suitable donor organs and is possible only through the profound generosity and altruism of those who are willing to donate or those who consent to donation on behalf of their loved ones. Thorough oversight of transplantation is performed at the national level, which is intended to ensure the best use of this precious resource.

REFERENCES

1. Program specific Reports. Registry of transplant recipients. Available at: http://www.srtr.org/csr/current/Centers/Default.aspx. Accessed June 2013.
2. OPTN data as of June 1, 2013. Available at: http://optn.transplant.hrsa.gov/latestData/viewDataReports.asp. Accessed May 31, 2013.
3. OPTN Bylaws. Available at: http://optn.transplant.hrsa.gov/policiesAndBylaws/bylaws.asp. Accessed May 31, 2013.
4. Centers for Medicare & Medicaid Services (CMS), HHS. Medicare Program; hospital Conditions of Participation: Requirements for approval and re-approval of transplant centers for perform organ transplants. Fed Regist 2007;72(61): 5197–280.
5. National Organ Transplant Act, 42, United States Code, Section 273 et seq 1987.
6. Department of Health and Human Services. Organ Procurement and Transplant Network: Final Rule. 42 CFR Section 121, 2005.
7. McDiamid SV, Pruett TL, Graham WK. The oversight of solid organ transplantation in the United States. Am J Transplant 2008;8:739–44.
8. Abecassis MM, Burke R, Cosimi AB, et al. Transplant center regulation– a mixed blessing? An ASTS Council viewpoint. Am J Transplant 2008;8:2496–502.
9. Hamilton TE. Regulatory oversight in transplantation: are the patients really better off? Curr Opin Organ Transplant 2013;18:203–9.
10. Schold J, Arrington CJ, Levine G. Significant alterations in reported clinical practice associated with increased oversight of organ transplant center performance. Prog Transplant 2010;20:279–87.

Allocation of Resources for Organ Transplantation

Praveen Kandula, MD[a], T. Anthony Anderson, MD, PhD[b],
Parsia A. Vagefi, MD, FACS[c],*

KEYWORDS

- Organ allocation • Organ transplantation • Wait list
- United Network for Organ Sharing
- Organ Procurement and Transplantation Network

KEY POINTS

- Organ allocation in the United States has developed into a highly regulated and efficient process over the last 6 decades.
- The process of organ allocation is a coordinated effort between organ procurement organizations, transplant centers, and the hospitals managing deceased donors.
- Continued refinement of regulations governing allocation are sought to optimize equitable allocation and patient outcomes.
- Despite these efforts, the greatest factor limiting organ transplantation remains the disparity between the number of donor organs available and the increasing wait-listed population.

INTRODUCTION

Therapeutic advances in surgical techniques, immunosuppression, and patient management have made transplantation of human organs a standard therapeutic option for the treatment of advanced organ failure. In the United States, currently more than 15,000 kidney, 5500 liver, 2000 heart, 1600 lung, and 200 pancreas transplants are performed annually (**Table 1**).[1] Most of these organs are derived from deceased donors, and their allocation becomes increasingly challenging in the setting of demand far outpacing supply. Policies have been established, and refined as needed, to make such allocation fair and equitable. As organs can be potentially transported

[a] Department of Medicine, Massachusetts General Hospital, Harvard Medical School, 55 Fruit Street, Boston, MA 02114, USA; [b] Department of Anesthesia, Massachusetts General Hospital, Harvard Medical School, 55 Fruit Street, Boston, MA 02114, USA; [c] Division of Transplant Surgery, Department of Surgery, Massachusetts General Hospital, Harvard Medical School, 55 Fruit Street, White 544b, Boston, MA 02114, USA
* Corresponding author.
E-mail address: pvagefi@partners.org

Anesthesiology Clin 31 (2013) 667–674
http://dx.doi.org/10.1016/j.anclin.2013.08.002   anesthesiology.theclinics.com

Table 1
Current number of patients on the UNOS waiting list and the number of patients transplanted in 2012 by organ[a]

Organ	Number on Wait List	Number Transplanted
Kidney	96,103	15,150
Liver	15,854	5757
Heart	3495	2169
Lung	1690	1622
Pancreas	1188	227

[a] Waiting list for each organ on April 19, 2013 and number transplanted in 2012.
Data from OPTN. Available at: http://optn.transplant.hrsa.gov/latestData/rptData.asp. Accessed April 24, 2013; and UNOS. Available at: http://transplantliving.org/?module=data&trend=transplants-organ-year&year=2012. Accessed April 24, 2013.

across the states, ordinances and oversight are provided federally by the US Department of Health and Human Services (HHS). A brief description of the history, as well as the methodologies involved in allocating these relatively scarce resources, are discussed here, with a focus on abdominal organ transplantation.

HISTORICAL PERSPECTIVE

On December 23, 1954, Dr Joseph Murray and Dr David Hume at Brigham Hospital in Boston performed the first successful transplant, a kidney, between identical twin brothers. Over the next 3 decades, successful deceased donor kidney, lung, pancreas, liver, and heart transplants followed. During this time, common law provided no one with clear property rights to human corpses. No institution had authority to sell or bequest a body or its parts. Only relatives were allowed to decide how to bury and dispose of a corpse. In 1968 the concept of a brain dead donor was formalized by an ad hoc committee at Harvard Medical School. They suggested revising the definition of death such that a subset of patients with a devastating neurologic injury would be suitable for organ donation under the dead donor rule.[2] As organ transplantation became possible, there was no legal system in place allowing individuals to donate their organs for transplant purposes after their death. In 1968, the Uniform Anatomical Gift Act (UAGA) was established which gave adults the right to donate their organs on death. By 1973, every state had adopted UAGA. However, although UAGA was clear about organ donation, it said nothing about sales. Some states had instituted laws that prohibited the sale of human bodies and organs before the UAGA; most were repealed afterward.[3,4]

Before 1984, deceased donor organs were procured and shared by several imprecisely coordinated private groups. In September 1983, Dr H. Barry Jacobs founded the International Kidney Exchange, Ltd in Virginia to broker human kidneys. Dr Jacobs, previously a practicing physician, had his Virginia license revoked in 1977 because of a mail fraud conviction involving Medicare and Medicaid, resulting in a 10-month prison sentence. In 1983, Dr Jacobs sent brochures to 7500 US hospitals offering his services. For a $2000 to $5000 commission, Dr Jacobs would find healthy individuals to sell a kidney for up to $10,000 to those in need of a transplant. Although legal when announced, within 6 months, Virginia passed a law to prohibit human organ sales. Several states followed with similar legislation.[5]

The National Organ Transplant Act (NOTA) was approved on October 19, 1984, and banned the buying and selling of organs in the United States. It was sponsored by

Representative Al Gore and Senator Orrin Hatch and amended in 1988 and 1990 to further define Organ Procurement Organization (OPO) oversight. NOTA created the Organ Procurement and Transplantation Network (OPTN), a nongovernmental organization, which maintained a national organ-matching registry. NOTA required that OPTN be managed by a private, nonprofit organization under federal contract. The United Network for Organ Sharing (UNOS) was awarded the national OPTN contract in 1986 by HHS. UNOS is the only organization that has ever operated OPTN. As part of the OPTN contract, UNOS must comply with transplant regulations and ensure that key fundamental policies are carried out (**Box 1**). UNOS members include patients with end-stage organ disease, transplanted patients, donor families, representatives of health, medical, and scientific groups, transplant centers, OPOs, and tissue typing laboratories. UNOS is governed by physicians and OPO professionals who are elected to their positions.[6]

The federal government provides significant oversight for organ transplantation and donation. In April 1998, HHS published a final directive requiring OPTN and UNOS to adopt new organ allocation guidelines. The Final Rule for Organ Procurement and Transplantation went into effect in March 2000 and further established the specific role and legal authority of OPTN.[7] The Final Rule altered the existing allocation system prioritizing national over local allocation. This was met with widespread criticism. Some states passed laws to limit transfer of organs out of state. The amended Final Rule, which finally went into effect, stated that organs should be distributed as widely as possible. In addition, OPTN responsibilities as mandated in the Final Rule included overseeing organ procurement policy compliance, equitable organ allocation, appropriate training of key medical staff, accumulating transplantation performance data, evaluating transplantation practices for HHS, and protecting public safety and health with regard to transplantation. OPTN has authority over transplant hospitals and organ procurement organizations but not over practitioners.[8] In May 2006, HHS published the Final Rule for Organ Procurement Organizations, which sets rigid performance measures and threatens loss of ability to procure and transplant organs if these measures are not met.[9]

The current UNOS organ allocation process involves 2 steps and combines information supplied by individual transplant teams with the UNOS criteria for organ transplantation. The initial step involves physicians deciding whether a patient requires a transplant and that patient's odds of survival and benefit after the transplant using clinical and psychosocial data. Whereas the clinical assessment evaluates the health of each potential organ recipient, the psychosocial evaluation assesses the patient's ability to handle the stress of the transplantation process and compliance with the burdensome lifelong posttransplant medical treatment. The second step of organ allocation involves the UNOS method of recipient selection from the wait list based on medical criteria, medical usefulness, and justice. Medical criteria include anatomic

---

Box 1
UNOS policies as part of the OPTN contract

1. Institute an organ-sharing organization that maximizes the efficient use of deceased organs through just and timely matching and allocation.

2. Establish a system to collect, evaluate, and publish information pertaining to the patient wait list, organ matching, and transplantation.

3. Guide persons and organizations via grants and contracts in order to increase the number of organs donors.

and immunologic compatibility between the donor and recipient organs, medical need for transplantation, and the efficient transport of the donor organ to minimize cold ischemic time and optimize organ viability and outcome. Critical factors involved in medical usefulness are achieving the longest possible patient survival, striving for considerable improvement in the patient's quality of life, as well as the cost-benefit ratio. Justice includes giving priority to patients with the most medical necessity, patients who have spent a greater time on the wait list, local access to organs for transplantation, and policies that prevent restricting access of patients to the transplant list.[10]

UNOS runs UNet, a computer network to link all OPOs and transplant centers, which transplant staff can access around the clock. DonorNet, a part of UNet, was launched in 2006 and allows more efficient matching and placement. The UNOS Organ Center assists in placing donated organs for transplantation, gathering donor information and matching donated organs to recipients, and assisting organ transportation. HHS and OPTN continue to advocate to increase the number of deceased donors as well as the average and total number of deceased donor organs transplanted. In addition, living donation has emerged as a secondary focus for OPTN as a result of the increasing need for organs.[11]

ALLOCATION
Regions, Donation Service Areas, and OPO

Through the oversight of the OPTN, the country is divided into 11 geographic regions (**Table 2**). Each region is further divided into several donation service areas (DSA) that are determined by regional population characteristics. Each DSA is served by an OPO. There are currently 58 regional OPOs that are required to be members of UNOS and follow their guidelines: 7 of the 58 are hospital based and the remaining 51 are independent. Each DSA can have only 1 OPO, but a single OPO can serve multiple DSAs. All transplant centers within a service area depend on the OPO to facilitate the organ donation process. OPOs are nonprofit organizations and are charged with the responsibility of facilitating the organ and tissue procurement process and distributing organs to centers within the areas they serve. Members of the OPO coordinate with hospital teams, family members of deceased donors, and coordinators for transplant centers to allow organ donation and transplantation to occur seamlessly in the shortest period

Table 2	
States in the 11 different regions	
Region 1	Connecticut, Maine, Massachusetts, New Hampshire, Rhode Island, Eastern Vermont
Region 2	Delaware, District of Columbia, Maryland, New Jersey, Pennsylvania, West Virginia, Northern Virginia
Region 3	Alabama, Arkansas, Florida, Georgia, Louisiana, Mississippi, Puerto Rico
Region 4	Oklahoma, Texas
Region 5	California, Nevada, New Mexico, Utah
Region 6	Alaska, Hawaii, Idaho, Montana, Oregon, Washington
Region 7	Illinois, Minnesota, North Dakota, South Dakota, Wisconsin
Region 8	Colorado, Iowa, Kansas, Missouri, Nebraska, Wyoming
Region 9	New York, Western Vermont
Region 10	Indiana, Michigan, Ohio
Region 11	Kentucky, North Carolina, South Carolina, Tennessee, Virginia

of time. Both OPOs and transplant centers are judged by their outcomes and have a common goal: the OPOs aim to maximize the number of organs procured and transplanted, and the transplant centers to achieve optimal patient outcomes.

Kidney Allocation

Kidneys are first allocated to candidates who are listed for dual organs, such as those in need of kidney-pancreas, kidney-liver, or kidney-heart transplant. As detailed later, in dual organ allocation, the allocation of the kidney allograft follows candidates based on priority listing for other organs. If there is no matched candidate for a dual or multi-organ transplant, then kidneys are allocated based on an end-stage renal disease patient's time on the waiting list, degree of HLA matching, degree of sensitization as determined by percent panel reactive antibodies, and age.

Kidney allocation follows a schema whereby organs procured within a region are usually first offered locally at the DSA level, before being offered regionally and nationally, largely based on the candidates duration on the transplant wait list. Perfectly matched kidneys, termed 0 (zero) antigen mismatched kidneys, are one of the exceptions to this algorithm; this refers to the donor and recipient being identical for HLA A, B, and DR antigens. ABO identical kidneys are first preferentially allocated to 0 antigen mismatched candidates, given improved outcomes within this cohort.[1] A 0 antigen mismatched kidney reflects an immunologic advantage in donor/recipient matching, rather than a true measure of the donor kidney allograft quality. If no one is identified, then allocation is considered for blood group compatible patients. For the purpose of allocation, blood group O is compatible with blood group B and blood group A is compatible with blood group AB. At each level, if more than 1 recipient is identified, then a point system is implemented to assist with allocation; the patient with the most points receives the kidney. Allocation of kidney points is based on several criteria including time on the wait list, pediatric recipient status, history of previous kidney donation, and so forth.

After allocation of a kidney to a candidate, and before the transplant proceeds, immune compatibility is further tested through cross-match testing; that is, in vitro testing of a potential recipient's blood sample with the deceased donor's cells. A population demonstrating increasing difficulty in achieving deceased donor renal transplant are the highly sensitized group of renal failure patients.[12] These patients, who represent nearly a third of kidney transplant candidates, demonstrate a heightened immune response to the donor despite being a blood type match. Sensitization usually occurs after blood transfusions, pregnancies, or from a previous transplanted organ. Although planned desensitization protocols have gained wider acceptance in living donor kidney transplantation, the unpredictable timing of deceased donor transplantation has made achieving desensitization in the candidate without a living donor more challenging.[13]

Although seemingly complex, the list of wait-listed candidates is maintained on computer servers and programs help in identifying the most suitable recipients first. When a deceased donor kidney becomes available, an offer is made to a transplant center through the OPO. Each transplant center has the option to accept or decline the kidney for their individual recipients. Each transplant center maintains its own list of transplant patients and must decide on the suitability of the donor for their potential recipients. If the offer is refused, the next patient on the wait list, either at the same center or at a different transplant center, is then evaluated as a potential recipient in the same manner. At each transplant center, there is a point of contact between the center and the OPO, and the transplant center is given 1 hour to make a decision to accept or refuse the kidney for that recipient. The complete donor information, as well as the ability to accept or decline the offered organ, is greatly facilitated through the web-based portal DonorNet. Although allocation of most organs occur before deceased donor procurement, kidney allocation can proceed after procurement given the extended cold ischemic time a kidney can tolerate (up to 36 hours). However, it should be noted that prolonged ischemic times can adversely affect graft function as demonstrated by higher rates of delayed graft function and the potential for inferior long-term graft survival.[14]

Pancreas Allocation

Pancreas allocation can proceed via multiple paths: (1) simultaneous kidney-pancreas allocation; (2) pancreas alone allocation; and less frequently (3) islet cell allocation. Generally, pancreas from donors aged less than 50 years and body mass index (BMI, calculated as weight in kilograms divided by the square of height in meters) less than 35 kg/m^2 are allocated for pancreas transplantation; the remainder are considered for islet cell transplantation or research. Pancreas allocation in large part follows similar rules of wait time, HLA mismatch, ABO compatibility, and degree of sensitization as for kidney allocation. Pancreata are first allocated for dual organ transplantation along with kidneys for patients with end-stage renal disease secondary to diabetes mellitus. If no suitable dual organ recipient is identified, the OPO can then pursue allocation of isolated pancreas grafts and isolated kidney grafts. On average, a pancreas graft can endure up to 12 hours of cold ischemic time.

Liver Allocation

Since 2002, liver allocation has been based on the model for end-stage liver disease (MELD) scoring system that was originally developed as a prognostic tool for patients undergoing transjugular intrahepatic portosystemic shunts (TIPS). It has been subsequently validated as an important tool predicting short-term mortality among patients awaiting liver transplantation.[15] MELD scores can range from 6 to 40, and are calculated for adults based on a formula incorporating the total bilirubin, internationalized normalized ratio (INR), and serum creatinine level. Its counterpart in children (<12 years) is the pediatric end-stage liver disease (PELD) score and differs from MELD in that it uses age, albumin, total bilirubin, and INR to calculate scores.

Adult deceased liver donors, similar to kidney donors, are offered locally first within the DSA of the OPO, followed by regional and then national offers. In contrast to kidney and pancreas allocation where wait time plays a significant role in determining a person's place on the wait list, liver candidates are ranked by the severity of their disease based on the MELD score calculation. There are instances when a patient may be listed as Status 1, that is, patients facing imminent death (<7 days) and in emergent need of a liver transplant, and thus these patients are given regional priority for liver allocation over all local candidates. Status 1 candidates include patients with acute fulminant liver failure (patients with the onset of encephalopathy within the previous 8 weeks and no history of liver abnormalities) and who are (1) ventilator dependent or (2) on dialysis or (3) with INR greater than 2; those with primary nonfunction or hepatic artery thrombosis within 7 days after transplant, and acute decompensated Wilson disease. MELD scores are updated ranging from yearly to every 7 days, depending on the severity of the liver disease; candidates with higher MELD scores are updated more frequently. Additional MELD points (termed MELD exception points) can be awarded for certain disease states in which the candidate's true MELD score fails to reflect the severity of their disease and thus their risk for death or wait-list dropout. Thus, for example, patients with hepatocellular carcinoma, portopulmonary hypertension, or hepatopulmonary syndrome are awarded additional MELD exception points every 3 months they remain on the wait list to allow their MELD score to increase and be in contention for deceased donor liver allocation. Mazzaferro and colleagues defined in 1996, the subset of patients with unresectable HCC for whom liver transplantation is the appropriate treatment, and thus developed the "Milan criteria". Transplantation within the Milan criteria (single tumor of 5 cm in diameter, or two to three tumors of 3 cm in diameter) resulted in overall and recurrence-free survival rates of 85% and 92%, respectively, at 4 years. Currently, only HCC patients within Milan criteria are allowed MELD exception points.[16] For adolescent and pediatric liver donors, allocation is preferentially directed to pediatric candidates first at the local, regional, and national levels before being considered for adult candidates. It should also be noted that liver allografts can endure a cold ischemic time of approximately 12 hours.

Dual Organ Allocation

Patients needing multiple organ transplants tend to be sicker and receive special allocation status. The most common organ transplanted as a part of combined organ transplantation is the kidney. Although a kidney allograft could be transplanted in combination with any organ, the most common scenarios include liver-kidney, pancreas-kidney, and heart-kidney transplant. In large part, allocation of the kidney follows the allocation of other major organs as needed.

SUMMARY

In the last several decades, a dynamic and highly regulated process of organ donation and subsequent allocation has developed. The organ allocation policy developed by UNOS was based on the consensus of transplant experts and balances justice and usefulness. Although the criteria are slightly different for each organ, generally organs are allocated to patients within the local OPO first, then regional patients, then nationally. The success of organ donation is facilitated by the work of many individuals representing governmental factions, the nonprofit sector, and a wide array of health care individuals associated with transplant centers and donor hospitals. The success of organ transplantation is now most limited by the inadequate supply of donor organs to meet the increasing needs of an expanding wait list population.

REFERENCES

1. OPTN: annual data report. Available at: http://optn.transplant.hrsa.gov/latestData/rptData.asp. Accessed April 24, 2013.
2. A definition of irreversible coma: report of the ad hoc committee of the Harvard Medical School to examine the definition of brain death. JAMA 1968;205:337–40.
3. Hurley JL. Cashing in on the transplant list: an argument against offering valuable compensation for the donation of organs. J High Tech Law 2004;117.
4. Hansmann H. The economics and ethics of markets for human organs. J Health Polit Policy Law 1989;14:57–85.
5. Denise SH. Regulating the sale of human organs. Va Law Rev 1985;71:1015–38.
6. Van Meter CH. The organ allocation controversy: how did we arrive here? Ochsner J 1999;1:6–11.
7. Weimer DL. Public and private regulation of organ transplantation: liver allocation and the final rule. J Health Polit Policy Law 2007;32:9–49.
8. McDiarmid SV, Pruett TL, Graham WK. The oversight of solid organ transplantation in the United States. Am J Transplant 2008;8:739–44.

9. Howard RJ, Cornell DL, Cochran L. History of deceased organ donation, transplantation, and organ procurement organizations. Prog Transplant 2012;22: 6–16 [quiz: 17].

10. Neuberger J. Rationing life-saving resources–how should allocation policies be assessed in solid organ transplantation. Transpl Int 2012;25:3–6.

11. Brown RS Jr, Higgins R, Pruett TL. The evolution and direction of OPTN oversight of live organ donation and transplantation in the United States. Am J Transplant 2009;9:31–4.

12. Jordan SC, Pescovitz MD. Presensitization: the problem and its management. Clin J Am Soc Nephrol 2006;1:421–32.

13. Alachkar N, Lonze BE, Zachary AA, et al. Infusion of high-dose intravenous immunoglobulin fails to lower the strength of human leukocyte antigen antibodies in highly sensitized patients. Transplantation 2012;94:165–71.

14. Irish WD, Ilsley JN, Schnitzler MA, et al. A risk prediction model for delayed graft function in the current era of deceased donor renal transplantation. Am J Transplant 2010;10(10):2279–86.

15. Saab S, Wang V, Ibrahim AB, et al. MELD score predicts 1-year patient survival post-orthotopic liver transplantation. Liver Transpl 2003;9:473–6.

16. Mazzaferro V, Regalia E, Doci R, et al. Liver transplantation for the treatment of small hepatocellular carcinomas in patients with cirrhosis. N Engl J Med 1996; 334:693–9.

Ethics of Transplantation

Antonia J. Cronin, MA, PhD, MRCP (UK)

KEYWORDS

- Organ donation and transplantation • Nonstandard organs for transplant
- Donor and donor organ quality • Transplantation-related research

KEY POINTS

- The contribution of landmark scientific discoveries to the enterprise and success of clinical transplantation has been invaluable, but they have not eliminated the significant variability in transplant outcomes related to donor organ quality prompted by the shortage of organs available for transplantation.
- Different types of donations, and nonstandard or expanded criteria donor organs that fail to meet standard criteria and are often associated with less good outcomes, are now being transplanted into selected recipients as a means of increasing the donor pool.
- The use of non-standard organs creates a number of potential ethical and legal problems in terms of consent and liability, and new challenges for research and service development.
- The challenge lies in developing a system of organ donation which responds to an evolving ethical landscape and continues to incorporate scientific innovation in order to adequately meet the needs of recipients, while at the same time safeguards the interests and autonomy of the donor.

INTRODUCTION

For almost 60 years research has made an invaluable contribution to the success of clinical transplantation. Landmark scientific discoveries include the description, development, and practical use of HLA tissue typing, understanding of the role of antibodies in hyperacute rejection, and the use and application of immunosuppressive treatment to prevent graft rejection.[1–6]

These and other advances have become a routine and integral part of health care service delivery, but they have not eliminated the significant variability in transplant outcomes related to donor organ quality, which have more recently been brought into focus by the shortage of organs available for transplantation. Organ shortage means that, in addition to standard deceased donor organs, nonstandard, expanded criteria, or marginal donor organs, which fail to meet standard criteria and are often

Disclosure: Dr A.J. Cronin is a member of the UK Donation Ethics Committee (UKDEC).
NIHR Biomedical Research Centre, Guy's and St Thomas' NHS Foundation Trust, MRC Centre for Transplantation, Guy's Hospital, King's College London, Fifth Floor Tower Wing, London SE1 9RT, UK
E-mail address: antonia.cronin@kcl.ac.uk

associated with less good outcomes, are now being transplanted into selected recipients as a means of increasing the donor pool.[7]

The standard criteria donor has no universally accepted definition, but standard donor status has usually been regarded as limited to organs donated from a heart-beating donor, aged between 10 and 50 years, after a diagnosis of brain death.[8,9] In the United Kingdom, this status is met after diagnosis and confirmation of brain-stem death.[10] In contrast in the United States, and many other countries, this status is met after a diagnosis of whole brain death, meaning the irreversible cessation of all brain function. The application of the concept of whole brain death in the context of deceased organ donation has long since been criticized and disputed, because most patients who are determined to be brain dead in the United States do not have loss of all brain function. For example, hypothalamic function may remain intact. For this and other reasons, there are increasing proposals to change the definition of brain death and abandon the so-called dead donor rule.[11–13] However, as regards the status of the donated organ, the fact that it has been retrieved from a heart-beating donor seems sufficient to justify its definition as standard.

The term expanded criteria donor (ECD) has been used since the early 1990s to describe donors and donor organs with various characteristics associated with poorer outcomes. The term has since been formally implemented into the US organ allocation scheme. A deceased donor kidney is considered to be an ECD organ if the estimated adjusted risk of graft failure is equal to or greater than 70% (relative risk$\geq$1.70) when compared with standard deceased donor kidneys. Characteristics that define an ECD kidney include age equal to or older than 60 years, or age 50 to 59 years plus 2 of the following: cerebrovascular accident as the cause of death, preexisting hypertension, or terminal creatinine greater than 1.5 mg/dL.[8,9] ECDs are a heterogeneous group. In this article, the term nonstandard donor (NSD) is used to refer to any donor who fails to meet standard criteria. Reports vary, but the consensus view is that as the donor's divergence from the standard description increases, so the likelihood of a successful transplant outcome reduces.

The nonstandard status of donor organs creates several potential problems in terms of medicolegal consent and liability. Furthermore, the distinction in clinical practice between standard and NSD transplants may produce unexpected legal effects that effectively inhibit the use of NSD organs. This has prompted an urgent need for clarification of the effect of using NSD organs in areas such as recipient and donor consent, liability for negligence, and the law of product liability.[7] Alongside this, nonstandard status has also created new challenges for research and service development. In particular, there is a need to identify ways to overcome the variability in transplant outcome related to nonstandard status and donor organ quality and optimize successful donation. Emerging experimental scientific evidence suggests that there are ways in which these barriers may be overcome and interventions to facilitate this are under development.[14–17] However, questions remain on the legitimacy of incorporating such interventions into clinical practice and the extent to which intervening and conducting research on the dying and the deceased in order to improve the lives of the living can be justified. For example, if such interventions are to be properly understood as an integral and necessary part of organ procurement, how are we to determine when an individual donor is really dead, or dead enough, for them to be incorporated? It is not clear that upholding the dead donor rule is always possible, nor yet a necessary part of the decision-making process, in these circumstances.

Some argue that the need for nonstandard organs results from society's failure to compel the retrieval of all suitable standard organs from the deceased as a community resource.[18,19] However, an increasing body of domestic and international law governing organ donation and transplantation expressly requires individual consent and authorization in the decision to donate.[20] Others seem to claim that the emphasis on meeting demand is misguided and suggest that without an exploration of the potential to reduce demand, particularly through prevention, it is not possible to validly defend supply-side initiatives that may involve reducing the protection of an individual's interests at the end of life.[21] Strategic health policy aimed at prevention of disease, for example diabetes, is without question worthwhile, but given that, for example, in Europe and the United States, as elsewhere, projected figures estimate a 50% increase in end-stage renal disease over the next 10 years, it seems unlikely that preventive measures alone will be able to overcome the untimely, and arguably unnecessary, loss of life as a result of organ failure that we are witnessing.[22–24] Several publicly funded initiatives have targeted prevention. Others have prompted an increase in the overall number of deceased donations.[25] Some countries have incorporated changes to existing legislation in an effort to increase the donation rates. For example, in the United States, the Uniform Anatomical Gift Act required request law mandates hospital personnel to discuss with the relative of a deceased patient the possibility of an anatomic gift. This Act is not in effect in all US states states. However, the federal and many state governments have passed legislation to make such requests compulsory.[26,27] Other countries have passed so-called presumed consent legislation.[28] However, it is generally acknowledged that there is no quick fix solution to the shortfall in organs available for transplantation, which, given the predicted estimates, seems likely to be here to stay. The challenge therefore lies in developing a strategy that responds to the evolving landscape and incorporates scientific innovation in order to adequately meet the needs of recipients, but at the same time safeguards donor autonomy.

IDEAL, STANDARD, AND NONSTANDARD ORGANS FOR TRANSPLANTS

The ideal donation, as was the case in the first successful transplant by Murray in 1954, is between young adult identical twins, whose genetic identity precludes any tissue incompatibility and whose kidneys are unaffected by deterioration related to age or hypertension.[29] No immunosuppression is required and indefinite graft survival should be achievable. It may seem obvious that only the best, that is genetically identical, organ should be offered to recipients. If the supply of such ideal donors were surplus to demand, there would be no need to use nonideal organs for transplants of any sort. However, monozygotic identity is uncommon, and moreover, since the early era, increased knowledge of transplant immunology and HLA tissue typing, along with the development of effective immunosuppression, has led to the much improved results from nonidentical (allograft) donors, which are typical of modern transplantation (In transplant terminology, a homo graft comes from oneself, an isograft from an identical individual, an allograft from a nonidentical human donor, and a xenograft comes from another species).

Reliable outcomes predictions, based on cumulative graft survivals, can now estimate success according to the type of donor.[30] The terms standard, expanded, and nonstandard have evolved in response to the need to balance clinical information about the predicted variability in the transplant outcome against the principle of equality of opportunity in access to donor organs to all those registered waiting on the national deceased donor transplant list.

The standard criteria donor has no universally accepted definition, but standard donor status has usually been regarded as limited to organs donated from a heart-beating donor, aged between 10 and 50 years, after a diagnosis of brain death.[8,9] An NSD, for instance an elderly donor, fails to meet these criteria and the consensus view is that, as the donor's divergence from the standard description increases, so the likelihood of a successful transplant outcome reduces. However, nonstandard status is not static. It is generally acknowledged that fewer people now die from catastrophic brain injury after road traffic accidents, and advances in hospital intensive care management have changed the context in which the diagnosis and confirmation of death are made. This situation has led to different types of donation taking place.[31,32] In particular, there has been a significant increase in the proportion of controlled donations after withdrawal of life-sustaining treatment and diagnosis of circulatory death (cDCD). At present in the United Kingdom, donation after circulatory death (DCD) is organ donation that takes place after diagnosis of death by cardiorespiratory criteria as laid down in the *Code of Practice for Diagnosis and Confirmation of Death*.[10] Because of previously reported inferior outcomes, donations after a diagnosis of circulatory death (formerly described as non–heart-beating donation) have usually been classified as nonstandard or expanded criteria.[30] However, several studies now suggest that under controlled intensive care conditions, the outcomes from DCD kidneys may equal those of standard donations.[33,34] DCD donations are a particularly important group because they have been responsible for a significant expansion of the donor pool in recent years. For example, in the United Kingdom, the 50% increase in donor numbers over the last 5 years reported recently was almost entirely accounted for by donations after the controlled withdrawal of life-sustaining treatment and diagnosis of circulatory death (cDCD).[30] Much medical, ethical, and legal discussion centers on the question of their reduced viability, as well as addressing ethical and legal issues specific to them. The importance of patient involvement in the decision-making process means that it remains relevant to consider them under the nonstandard or expanded criteria heading.

The most successful transplants, which are mainly those coming from standard donors, achieve 80%, or more, 3-year cumulative graft survival. However, there is a sequence of success, headed by live identical twin donations, followed by other live, and then deceased, donations.[30,35] Next in the order of outcomes come NSD or ECD deceased donations, which are also sometimes referred to as marginal. Donors older than 60 years of age are invariably classified as nonstandard. Cassini and colleagues[36] have reported a significant negative effect of donor age on transplant survival and urge caution on the use of older donors. Others, for example Foss and colleagues,[37] have, in contrast, suggested that the clinical disadvantage of the nonstandard status of older donors is reduced if their kidneys go to recipients of the same age or older. Other varied negative donor factors, such as a history of neoplasia, hepatitis, behavioral risk factors, and ABO blood group compatibility, are common reasons for classifying donor organs as expanded criteria or nonstandard.[38–41] These NSD organs have become an important resource. It may seem inappropriate to encourage their use, because, by definition, their inferior outcomes may lead to a patient's early reinstatement on the transplant waiting list, immunologically sensitized and effectively more difficult to retransplant. However, against this situation must be set the evidence that, although inferior to standard donor organs, NSD organs do offer a potential benefit to the recipient. The alternatives are life on dialysis, which is usually (although not invariably) of lower quality, or death on the waiting list.[42] Thus, the acceptance and use of nonideal or NSD organs in clinical practice seems justified by their relatively beneficial effect and availability, which may offer the best, or only, opportunity for many waiting patients.

INTERVENTIONS TO OPTIMIZE SUCCESSFUL DONATION AND TRANSPLANTATION

Mason and Laurie[43] have perceptively noted the marked distinction in the public mind between the concept of tissue retention for, sometimes undefined, research purposes and that of organ donation and transplantation, for which, evidence suggests, support is significant. Nonstandard organs for transplantation, in particular organs donated after controlled withdrawal of treatment and confirmation of death by circulatory criteria, present an immediate challenge to this distinction. A prolonged withdrawal, or agonal, period is an important cause of decreased organ viability. The acceptance and use of nonstandard organs have prompted an urgent need to facilitate both interventions and research aimed at optimizing their successful donation and improving transplant outcomes. It has also increased calls to reconsider the dead donor rule.[11–13,44]

It has been reported that several interventions can improve the viability of nonstandard organs, and in particular, the viability of organs donated after the withdrawal of life-sustaining treatment and confirmation of death by circulatory criteria. These interventions include continuation of life-sustaining treatments, including respiratory support, intravenous fluids, and preexisting medication.[45] More invasive pharmacologic and mechanical interventions can also be used to improve donor organ quality. Examples include the administration of heparin to prevent blood clots forming in donor organs, insertion of arterial catheters to infuse preserving solutions, normothermic perfusion, and mechanical ventilation and cardiac compression (sometimes referred to in this context as resuscitation) in order to oxygenate donor organs, thereby preventing organ damage through lack of oxygen supply. Although evidence supporting these interventions is patchy, they have improved organ quality and transplant outcome in some studies. Their successful use in the United States has been reported.[14,46] Their use in the United Kingdom is currently limited by guidance published by the Department of Health.[47]

In general, if, in the context of patient treatment, compelling evidence emerged that a proposed intervention would significantly improve the outcome, it would be difficult for clinicians not to support or sanction its use. However, if, in the context of organ donation, similarly compelling evidence emerged that it was possible for some intervention or another to restore an otherwise nonstandard organ to standard organ status and improve the likelihood of successful donation, the responsibility incumbent on clinicians to support or sanction its use would be less clear. This is because such interventions do not offer any immediate benefit to the donor. The unique context of organ donation, specifically the requirement of altruistic donation and the idea of a gift relationship intended to benefit others, makes matters less straightforward.

There is no consensus view on whether such interventions should be considered as an integral part of donation or whether they are different actions requiring a different type of consent. In the United Kingdom, as elsewhere, these interventions, some of which are part of a program of research, have prompted concern about the protection of the individual donor's autonomy and interests.[48] Specifically, there is argument as to whether, and if so to what extent, an individual's decision to donate can, and properly should, be understood to incorporate their wish to donate organs in as good condition as possible and their willingness to consent to a range of interventions aimed at achieving this goal.

Such interventions are not intended to have, nor do they have, any therapeutic purpose or medical benefit for the donor. Moreover, they might even physically harm the donor. Even although the donor is approaching death, the possibility (even if remote) that the interventions might cause harm cannot be ignored. For instance, an intervention such as the administration of heparin may prompt a catastrophic intracerebral bleed and expedite a potential donor's death. Without the donor's, or their authorized representative's, prior consent, such an intervention would be illegal. However, if the consent process for donation included agreement to interventions, such as the administration of heparin, then their use in this context would be lawful.[49] It is therefore important to consider the potential advantage of the interventions to the transplant recipient against their potential to cause harm to the donor. The difficulty lies in being able to accurately ascertain what the wishes and therefore best interests of the donor would have been, and to determine which types of interventions they would have been be prepared to accept, or perhaps reject, as part of their decision to consent to donation. A further difficulty lies in being able to determine the point at which the donor's wishes are no longer relevant and the wishes of the potential recipient of an organ should take precedence.

Best Interests and Overall Benefit

Most potential donors are deeply unconscious both before and during the agonal period. This dilemma therefore cannot be resolved by active donor. In this setting, in the United States, the consent of the donor's family or representatives assumes an important role. However, in contrast, in the United Kingdom, the consent of relatives or nominated representatives cannot be invoked, because, under UK law, these individuals gain authority to consent to donation only after death has occurred.[50] In addition, neither advance decisions[51] nor lasting powers of attorney[52] are relevant because, under UK law, they confer authority only to refuse specific treatments and do not in themselves grant any powers of consent to organ donation or premortem intervention. However, because unconsciousness does involve mental incapacity, it may be possible to gain legal justification for such interventions on the grounds that they are in the donor's best interests.[53,54] In the United Kingdom, the best interests test is set out in the Mental Capacity Act (2005). The test obliges clinical decision makers to consider so far as is reasonably possible to ascertain:

1. The person's past and present wishes and feelings
2. The beliefs and values that would be likely to influence their decision if they had capacity
3. The other factors that they would be likely to consider if they were able to do so.[55]

The Mental Capacity Act Code of Practice emphasizes the importance of considering a person's social, emotional, cultural, and religious interests in determining what course of action may be in their best interests.[56]

In its report *An Ethical Framework for Controlled Donation after Circulatory Death*, the UK Donation Ethics Committee (UKDEC) uses the term best interests only in the context of specific legislation, in which the term has particular meaning. UKDEC otherwise uses the term overall benefit, which incorporates an assessment of best interests, when describing the course of action most appropriate to a particular patient at a particular time. The term overall benefit can be usefully applied to other jurisdictions when considering the balance of factors in the decision-making process in the end-of-life care pathway.[57]

The critical point in this care pathway, regardless of whether an individual patient may go on to become an organ donor, is the decision about whether further life-sustaining treatment is of overall benefit to them. If it has been established that further treatment is no longer of overall benefit to an individual and it has been further established that donation would be consistent with that individual's wishes, feelings, beliefs, and values, then it becomes relevant to consider and assess the legitimacy of interventions and research to optimize their donation.

Balancing Harm and Benefit

In their ethical framework, UKDEC sets out an approach to determining the course of action appropriate for a patient who lacks capacity in this context. Such a course of action requires an assessment to be made of whether the options available may cause, or risk causing, harm to the patient, the donor. In this context, harm encompasses 2 elements. One is the undesirable physical effect that may be caused by an intervention, such as the risk of unpleasant side effects of a medication, pain, discomfort, or distress. Potential physical harm may also include shortening, or perhaps extending, a patient's life and worsening their medical condition. The other is the harm that may be caused by doing wrong to the patient, such as by ignoring their expressed wishes for end-of-life care (see section 1.4.3 in Ref.[57]). So, when considering whether a particular intervention or course of action may cause harm to a patient, both of these elements need to be considered and a judgment made. The degree of harm inevitably varies with different interventions. The key recommendation is that clinicians should take account of this situation in order to reach a balanced view of the risk of harm when considering particular interventions or courses of action, encompassing both the risk of physical harm and the risk of doing wrong by not acting in accordance with the patient's wishes (see section 1.4 recommendation in Ref.[57]).

UKDEC has set out a spectrum of overlapping possibilities. It includes (1) donors who have both consented to donation and agreed to undergo any procedures that would increase the probability of a successful transplant; (2) donors who have simply consented to donation by joining the Organ Donation Register, signing a donor card or advanced directive; and (3) donors who have consented to donation (communicated by a third party, usually their family) without performing one of the formalities in (2). In addition, the third party category also includes (4) donors for whom consent is provided by their wishes and feelings; (5) donors for whom consent is provided by their beliefs and values that would be likely to influence their decision; and (6) donors for whom consent is provided although there is little or no evidence of their wishes and beliefs on donation, or for whom donation would be consistent with their beliefs and values (see section 1.4.8 in Ref.[57]).

It is important to decipher the difference between decisions made after a patient's death, which may not reflect the patient's wishes or be in accordance with their interests (category (6) above), versus decisions made about a patient's end-of-life care, which must be for the overall benefit of that patient. The stronger the evidence of the patient's desire to become an organ donor, the greater the weight this should be given in assessing whether a particular intervention would be of overall benefit to them. However, as UKDEC asserts, there can be no single standard test of overall benefit (see section 1.4.12 in Ref.[57]). Determining the overall benefit requires a nuanced approach that takes account of individual feelings, beliefs, and values alongside medical needs and consideration of the possible risks and burdens to the patient.

In recent draft guidance, UKDEC supports the view that in relation to a particular intervention, a clear justification for the intervention in terms of its potential to optimize donor organ quality and improve transplant outcomes should be identified. The absolute minimum level of intervention should be used consistent with facilitating the success of the transplant. When there is genuine uncertainty about whether an intervention has the potential to optimize donor organ quality and improve transplant outcomes, clinical research, where possible, should be undertaken. UKDEC has speculated that it seems likely that for a wide range of minor interventions, the potential benefits of the proposed interventions are likely to outweigh any potential harms that cannot be prevented or alleviated. If so, the proposed intervention would be of overall benefit to the donor. However, a few interventions will carry such serious risks of harm that strong evidence of the potential benefits will be needed in order for them to be of overall benefit to the donor.[58]

The draft guidance by UKDEC has gone further and usefully divided premortem interventions into 2 categories:

1. Those that are integral to the withdrawal of life-sustaining treatment, for example extubation or sedation
2. Those that are independent of the withdrawal of life-sustaining treatment (eg, femoral cannulation or the administration of intravenous heparin)[58]

This classification may provide a useful guide for clinicians in determining the most appropriate course of action for an individual patient.

It is crucial that, over time, this type of guidance is developed into a highly detailed and empirically informed resource, which can provide specific guidance on the issues highlighted and can be applied more generally.

NSD ORGANS: RECIPIENT CONSENT AND LIABILITY

The development of the expanded criteria into a separate nonstandard category of transplant, albeit seemingly beneficial, raises questions over the legitimacy of recipient consent and liability. If a nonstandard organ is transplanted without the recipient being made aware of its possible substandard status, it might be possible to bring an action for battery or trespass against the person, on the grounds that failure to inform the recipient of the organ's nature had vitiated their consent. However, in the absence of fraud or dishonesty, this is an unlikely proceeding. When a patient is aware, in broad terms, of the nature of a treatment (eg, that it is a transplant operation), the appropriate remedy seems more likely to be an action in negligence for failing to disclose its risks.[59]

It might be argued that to use a nonstandard treatment with an inferior outcome is prima facie negligent in itself. However, this argument can easily be rebutted in the context of organ donation and transplantation, in which nonstandard organs are offered as a valuable resource and are often superior to the alternatives available.

However, judicial decisions do emphasize the importance of individual autonomy and the need for a patient to be sufficiently informed to make a rational decision about any proposed treatment.[60] Withholding relevant information is unacceptable, regardless of whether the health care professional would condone it as being in the patient's interest.[61] To avoid liability, it seems essential to disclose the relative risks of nonstandard organs to all potential recipients. Because transplants occur at unpredictable times, and often at short notice, a discussion in advance is helpful. However, given the variability of nonstandard organs, it is unlikely that any prior discussion would be able to satisfy all the requirements of consent, and so a further discussion will be necessary at the time of operation. Most of this discussion will concern the specific nature of the organ on offer (eg, the age and comorbidity of the donor) and the likely outcome of the transplant operation. Information regarding the interventions already undertaken, or to be undertaken, to optimize successful donation will also be relevant. It will be particularly important to inform the potential recipient about any further interventions to be made after allocation but before transplantation (eg, infusion of preservation fluid as part of a program of research to improve graft outcome). Negligence in this context need not be confined to the transplanting doctors and research workers. Laboratory staff, donating hospital teams, donor medical advisers, and even lay donor representatives could also become liable for failure to provide information that would detract from the quality of the deceased's organs.[62,63] In such cases, protection of donor anonymity seems less important than the recipient's right of action.[64]

Early loss or deterioration of an NSD kidney implanted without adequately informed consent might at first sight seem to justify compensation for negligence. However, the issues are more complex. The recipient would have to show first, that the kidney would not have been accepted if its NSD status had been understood and second, that the inferior outcome stemmed from this status and not some other cause, such as disease recurrence, drug toxicity, or poor compliance.[65] If this situation is established, the extent of damage is assessable by comparison with the predicted outcome of a standard organ. However, damage requires to be proved. Early failure would not inevitably be the result of this consent-related negligence; some NSD kidneys have been shown to survive for more than 40 years.[66] If early failure does not occur, proof of causation and damage will become increasingly difficult to establish, unless the courts are prepared to accept clinical predictions of graft failure, which has not yet occurred. When assessing exacerbation of medical risks, judicial precedents seem to accept evidence based on estimation of the probable percentage increase in risk, which may point the way in NSD cases, although no such action has been brought.[67] The fact that NSD graft survival at 3 to 5 years after transplant is only 10% to 20% inferior to standard donor survival suggests some of the difficulties involved. However, similar problems have been resolved in other areas of medicolegal negligence.[61] Transplantation, from being a form of rescue procedure, in which high complication rates were expected and tolerated, has evolved into a mainstream medical treatment, in which negligent management may fairly be expected to compensate for its undesired consequences.

Finally, if an individual potential recipient is entitled to reject an organ from medical information that it does not meet standard criteria, why should they not also be allowed to reject an organ from an individual based on some other criteria, for example an individual donor's social circumstances, their race, cultural heritage, or any arbitrary reason? Suppose, for example, that a recipient chooses to refuse an offered organ because it had been disclosed that the donor was involved in criminal activity. The refusal of a life-saving donation on such a basis may to some seem unreasonable. However, if upholding a recipient's autonomy in the decision-making process to accept or reject an organ is to take precedence, it is unclear why some decisions should be more equal than others. Our goal perhaps should be to uphold transparency and individual autonomy and safeguard against inappropriate discrimination and the danger of thereby tarnishing the whole enterprise of transplantation. Experience gained from directed and conditional donation may provide a useful guide.

SUMMARY

The emergent acceptance and use of nonstandard expanded criteria organs for transplants has raised new questions, which have hitherto not been much considered. They now occupy an important place in organ donation and transplantation. Overall, the use of NSDs seems to be clinically acceptable, as being superior to dialysis or death on the waiting list, and ethically justifiable as a pragmatic response to prevailing public attitudes. Their eventual role remains unclear. It will depend on developments in clinical science and whether these and other interventions can legitimately be incorporated into the deceased organ donation and transplantation pathway. Developing a strategy that responds to the evolving ethical and legal landscape and incorporates scientific innovation in order to adequately meet the needs of recipients, but which safeguards donor autonomy, is essential.

Dr Antonia J. Cronin acknowledges that the research was funded/supported by the National Institute for Health Research (NIHR) Biomedical Research Center based at Guy's & St Thomas' National Health Service (NHS) Foundation Trust and King's College London. The views expressed are those of the author and not necessarily those of the NHS, the NIHR, or the Department of Health.

REFERENCES

1. Terasaki PI, McClelland JD. Microdroplet assay of human serum cytotoxins. Nature 1964;204:998–1000.
2. Van Rood JJ, Van Leeuwen A. Leucocyte grouping: a method and its application. J Clin Invest 1963;42:1382.
3. Van Rood JJ. Tissue typing and organ transplantation. Lancet 1969;1: 1142–6.
4. Patel R, Terasaki PI. Significance of the positive crossmatch test in kidney transplantation. N Engl J Med 1969;280:735–9.
5. Calne RY, White DJ, Thiru S, et al. Cyclosporin A in patients receiving renal allografts from cadaver donors. Lancet 1978;2:1323–7.
6. Starzl TE, Todo S, Fung J, et al. FK506 for human liver, kidney and pancreas transplantation. Lancet 1989;2:1000–4.
7. Cronin AJ, Douglas JF. Non-standard kidneys for transplants: clinical margins, medical morality, and the law. Med Law Rev 2013. http://dx.doi.org/10.1093/medlaw/fwt015.
8. United Network of Organ Sharing (UNOS) definition. Available at: http://www.unos.org/. NHS Blood and Transplant in the United Kingdom have not set out a definition. Accessed August 21, 2013.
9. Meier-Kreische HK, Cole EH, Schold JD, et al. Analysis of the expanded criteria donor kidneys: how good is you ECD going to be? Am J Transplant 2004; 4(Suppl 8):305.
10. A code of practice for the diagnosis and confirmation of death, Academy of Medical Royal Colleges of the United Kingdom (AOMRC). Available at: http://www.aomrc.org.uk/publications/statements/doc_view/42-a-code-of-practice-for-the-diagnosis-and-confirmation-of-death.html. Accessed August 21, 2013.
11. Fost N. Reconsidering the dead donor rule: is it important that organ donors be dead? Kennedy Inst Ethics J 2004;14(3):249–60.
12. Fost N. The unimportance of death. In: Arnold R, Schapiro R, Youngner S, editors. Defining death in a technologic age. Baltimore (MD): Johns Hopkins Press; 1999. p. 161–78.
13. Halevy A, Brody B. Brain death: reconciling definitions, criteria, and tests. Ann Intern Med 1993;119:519–25.
14. Boglione MM, Morandini MA, Barrenechea ME, et al. Pre-arrest heparinization and ventilation during warm ischemia preserves lung function in non-heart-beating donors. J Pediatr Surg 1999;34(12):1805–9.
15. Inokawa H, Date H, Okazaki M, et al. Effects of postmortem heparinization in canine lung transplantation with non-heart-beating donors. J Thorac Cardiovasc Surg 2005;129(2):429–34.
16. Okazaki M, Date H, Inokawa H, et al. Optimal time for post-mortem heparinization in canine lung transplantation with non-heart-beating donors. J Heart Lung Transplant 2006;25(4):454–60.

17. Sugimoto R, Date H, Sugimoto S, et al. Post-mortem administration of urokinase in canine lung transplantation from non-heart-beating donors. J Heart Lung Transplant 2006;25(9):1148–53.
18. Harris J. Organ procurement: dead interests, living needs. J Med Ethics 2003; 29:130–4.
19. Cronin AJ, Harris J. Authorisation, altruism and compulsion in the organ donation debate. Journal of Medical Ethics 2010;36(10):627–31.
20. The Human Tissue Act (2004) in England, Wales and Northern Ireland, The Human Tissue (Scotland) Act (2006) in Scotland. See also various forms of Uniform Anatomical Gift Act in the United States.
21. Garwood-Gowers A. Book review of Farrell AM, Price D and Quigley M, editors, organ shortage: ethics, law and pragmatism. Cambridge (UK): Cambridge University Press; 2011. http://dx.doi.org/10.1093/medlaw/fwt020. Published in Medical Law Review 2013.
22. UK Department of Health Figures. 2013. Available at: http://www.diabetes.org.uk/Documents/Reports/State-of-the-Nation-2012.pdf. Accessed August 21, 2013.
23. World Health Organization publication figures. Available at: http://www.who.int/mediacentre/factsheets/fs236/en/. Accessed August 21, 2013.
24. NHS Bloods and Transplant published figures for 2012. Available at: http://www.organdonation.nhs.uk/statistics/transplant_activity_report/current_activity_reports/ukt/activity_report_2011_12.pdf. Accessed August 21, 2013.
25. Organ Donation Taskforce (UK Government 2008) and NHS Blood and Transplant (2008-2013) media campaigns. Available at: http://www.organdonation.nhs.uk/campaigns/. Accessed August 21, 2013.
26. The Uniform Anatomical Gift Act (1968) and its various revisions.
27. Whyte KP, Selinger E, Caplan AL, et al. Nudge, nudge or shove, shove-the right way for nudges to increase the supply of donated cadaver organs. Am J Bioeth 2012;12(2):32–9.
28. Rithalia A, McDaid C, Suekarran S, et al. Impact of presumed consent for organ donation on donation rates: a systematic review. BMJ 2009;338:a3162.
29. Murray JE, Merrill JP, Harrison JH, et al. Kidney transplantation between seven pairs of identical twins. Ann Surg 1958;148:343–57.
30. Data are available from NHS Blood and Transplant, activity reports. Available at: http://www.organdonation.nhs.uk/ukt/statistics/transplant_activity_report/transplant_activity_report.jsp. Accessed January 14, 2013.
31. Murphy PG, Bodenham AR, Thompson JP. Diagnosis of death and organ donation in 2012. Br J Anaesth 2012;108(Suppl 1):1–2.
32. Price D. End-of-life treatment of potential organ donors: paradigm shifts in intensive and emergency care. Med Law Rev 2011;19:86.
33. Summers DM, Johnson RJ, Allen J, et al. Analysis of factors that affect outcome after transplantation of kidneys donated after cardiac death in the UK: a cohort study. Lancet 2010;376(9749):1303–11.
34. Summers DM, Johnson RJ, Hudson A, et al. Effect of donor age and cold storage time on outcome in recipients of kidneys donated after circulatory death in the UK: a cohort study. Lancet 2013;381(9868):727–34.
35. Port FK, Dykstra DM, Merion RM, et al. Trends and results for organ donation and transplantation in the United States 2004. Am J Transplant 2005;5:843.
36. Cassini MF, Cologna AJ, Tucci S Jr, et al. Why not to use kidneys from elderly donors. Transplant Proc 2010;42(2):417–20.
37. Foss A, Heldal K, Scott H, et al. Kidneys from deceased donors more than 75 years perform acceptably after transplantation. Transplantation 2009;87:1437–41.

38. Kauffman HM, Cherikh WS, McBride MA, et al. Deceased donors with a past history of malignancy: an Organ Procurement and Transplant Network/United Network for Organ Sharing Update. Transplantation 2007;84:272–4.

39. Punnett AS, McCarthy LJ, Dirks PB, et al. Patients with primary brain tumours as organ donors: case report and review of the literature. Pediatr Blood Cancer 2004;43(1):73–7.

40. Lo CM, Fan ST, Liu CL, et al. Safety and outcome of hepatitis B core antibody-positive donors in right-lobe living-donor liver transplantation. Liver Transpl 2003;9:827–32.

41. O'Connor KJ, Delmonico FL. Increasing the supply of kidneys for transplantation. Semin Dial 2005;18(6):460–2.

42. Schol J, Srinivas TR, Sehgal AR, et al. Half of kidney transplant candidates who are older than 60 years now placed on the waiting list will die before receiving a deceased-donor transplant. Clin J Am Soc Nephrol 2009;4:1239–45.

43. Mason JK, Laurie GT. Non-heart beating donation. In: Mason JK, Laurie GT, editors. Mason and McCall Smith's law and medical ethics. 8th edition. Oxford (United Kingdom): Oxford University Press; 2011. p. 549.

44. Joffe AR, Carcillo J, Anton N, et al. Donation after cardiocirculatory death: a call for a moratorium pending full public disclosure and fully informed consent. Philos Ethics Humanit Med 2011;6:17.

45. Bernat JL, D'Alessandro AM, Port FK, et al. Report of a national conference on donation after cardiac death. Am J Transplant 2006;6:281–91 This conference explored many controversies regarding determination of death after circulatory arrest, prerecovery donor management and use of pharmacological agents, donor eligibility, and outcomes.

46. Mason DP, Thuita L, Alster JM, et al. Should lung transplantation be performed using donation after cardiac death? The United States experience. J Thorac Cardiovasc Surg 2008;136:1061–6.

47. UK Department of Health. Legal issues relevant to non-heart-beating donation. 2009. Available at: https://www.gov.uk/government/uploads/system/uploads/attachment_data/file/138313/dh_109864.pdf. Accessed August 21, 2013.

48. Coggon J, Brazier M, Murphy P, et al. Best interests and potential organ donors. BMJ 2008;336:1346.

49. Bell MD. Emergency medicine, organ donation and the Human Tissue Act. Emerg Med J 2006;23:824–7.

50. Human Tissue Act (2004) sections 3–5, and Human Tissue (Scotland) Act 2006 Section 6–9 and 16.

51. Mental Capacity Act 2005 Section 24.

52. Mental Capacity Act 2005 Sections 16 and 17.

53. Mental Capacity Act 2005, section 1(5).

54. The Adults with Incapacity (Scotland) Act 2000.

55. Mental Capacity Act 2005, section 4(6).

56. Mental Capacity Act 2005 Code of Practice section 5. Available at: http://webarchive.nationalarchives.gov.uk/+/http:/www.justice.gov.uk/docs/mca-cp.pdf. Accessed August 21, 2013.

57. UK Donation Ethics Committee. An ethical framework for controlled donation after circulatory death. 2011. Available at: www.aomrc.org.uk/publications/reports-guidance/doc_download/9450-an-ethical-framework-for-controlled-donation-after-circulatory-death.html. Accessed August 21, 2013.

58. UKDEC Draft Guidance on premortem interventions to optimize donor organ quality and improve transplant outcomes in DCD, presented at a consensus

meeting on March 1, 2013, Royal College of Paediatrics and Child Health. London.

59. Chatterton v Gerson [1981] QB 432, [1981] 1 All ER 257.
60. Sidaway v Board of Governors of the Bethlem Royal Hospital [1985] AC 871; Pearce v United Bristol Healthcare Trust (1999) 48 BMLR 118.
61. Chester v Afshar [2005] 1 AC 134.
62. This has become more important in the United Kingdom after the transposition of the EU Organ Directive into domestic UK law. Directive of the European Council and Parliament on standards of quality and safety of human organs intended for transplantation. Directive 2010/53/EC of 7 July 2010; Human Tissue (The Quality and Safety of Organs for Transplantation) Regulations 2012 laid before Parliament for approval under Schedule 2 to the European Communities Act 1972.
63. Cronin AJ, Douglas JF, Sacks SH. Licensed to transplant: UK overkill on EU directive provides golden opportunity for research. J Med Ethics 2012;38: 593–5.
64. AB v Scottish Blood Transfusion Service [1990] SLR 263 – it was so found by a Scottish court in a case of a claim against a blood donor.
65. Bolam v Friern Hospital Management Committee [1957] 2 All ER 118.
66. Douglas JF, Craig WJ. Long-term survival after renal transplantation. In: Cecka MJ, Terasaki PI, editors. Clinical transplants. Los Angeles (CA): UCLA Immunogenetics Centre; 2010. p. 133–9.
67. Hotson v East Berkshire Area Health Authority [1987] 2 All ER, HL; Gregg v Scott [2005] UKHL 2.

Patient Selection and Preoperative Evaluation for Transplant Surgery

James Y. Findlay, MB, ChB, FRCA

KEYWORDS

- Solid-organ transplantation • Kidney transplantation • Liver transplantation
- Pretransplant evaluation • Patient selection • Preoperative testing
- Coronary artery disease

KEY POINTS

- All patients considered for abdominal organ transplantation undergo a pretransplant evaluation that screens for conditions known to influence posttransplant outcome and that may need pretransplant intervention or may influence transplant candidacy.
- In all abdominal transplant candidates, coronary artery disease (CAD) is prevalent and should be screened for, although the best algorithms and subsequent management are controversial.
- In liver transplant candidates, the portal hypertension associated syndromes of portopulmonary hypertension and hepatopulmonary syndrome (HPS) should be screened for.
- Patients with acute liver failure (ALF) undergo an evaluation process different from those with chronic liver failure. Cerebral edema and critical illness are particular concerns in this group.
- There is little good evidence to guide the identification of the patient who is too sick for transplant; cases should be decided on an individual basis after multidisciplinary discussion.

INTRODUCTION

During recent years, organ transplant has become a more frequently performed procedure. In 2010, more than 100,000 solid-organ transplants were performed worldwide, with a yearly increase of around 2%.[1] The most frequently transplanted organ is kidney; in 2010, at least 73,000 kidney transplants were performed in a total of 95 countries; for liver, the second most frequent, the figure was more than 21,500.[1] In countries with established transplant programs, the increase in transplant activity is

Department of Anesthesiology and Critical Care Medicine, Mayo Clinic, 200 First Street SW, Rochester, MN 55905, USA
E-mail address: findlay.james@mayo.edu

Anesthesiology Clin 31 (2013) 689–704
http://dx.doi.org/10.1016/j.anclin.2013.09.002   **anesthesiology.theclinics.com**

being outstripped by the number of people on the waiting list for transplant; for example, in the United States, the number of kidney transplants increased from approximately 14,000 in 2001 to 16,800 in 2011, whereas the number on the waiting list increased from 45,000 to more than 95,000 during the same period.[2,3] This discrepancy is driven on the demand side by an expansion in both the indications for organ transplant and an expansion of the range of patients for whom the procedure is considered appropriate, such as the old patient and those with more, or more severe comorbidities. On the supply side, there is a limited resource of available organs, which has not increased to meet demand despite efforts to increase availability by the use of living donors and the use of organs from less-than-ideal donors—"expanded criteria donors." In addition to the wait-listed patients, there are those who are considered for transplant but do not go on to be candidates because of a variety of reasons. All these patients undergo a pretransplant evaluation, including an assessment of the risk associated with undergoing the procedure, the results of which are part of the assessment of the patent's suitability as a transplant candidate. The anesthesiologist working in a transplant program is thus faced with making decisions not only on risk stratification and mitigation for a pretransplant patient but also that may influence the patient's candidacy for transplant. This role has become part of the regulatory framework: the United Network for Organ Sharing, which oversees organ allocation in the United States, requires that for liver transplant programs a Director of anesthesiology is appointed one of whose roles is to be involved in the selection process.[4]

Another aspect that is particular to most transplant patients is that the initial evaluation frequently occurs a considerable time before the actual transplant. In the United States, the median time between listing and transplant for kidney patients is currently around 3 years, for liver around 1 year.[3] In this time, considerable changes in a patient's condition may occur, either with regard to the underlying disease (for liver) or of comorbid conditions.

Most transplant procedures are not elective. An organ becomes available and must be transplanted within a limited time frame after recovery to remain viable. The potential recipient may have to travel to the medical facility, which limits the time available for investigation and treatment of any unexpected issues, making adequate initial evaluation and appropriate subsequent follow-up important. It is also important to be able to access the necessary information in a timely manner.

Each organ failure for which transplant is carried out has its unique precipitants and comorbidities; also, common comorbidities may have different implications depending on the organ to be transplanted, for example, the implications of CAD in a kidney transplant candidate are different from those in a liver transplant candidate. The transplant surgeries themselves vary significantly in complexity and potential for hemodynamic instability: consider a kidney transplant versus a liver transplant. Each organ has different supply/demand considerations, as well as consequences if a transplant is not performed (regardless of long-term outcomes, there are replacement therapies for kidney and pancreatic failure; there is none for liver failure). For these reasons, each organ has its own literature and the major part of this review reflects this. Cardiopulmonary issues are the most important for abdominal transplant and have generated considerable research and controversy; these issues are the focus of this review. There are, of course, many other associated conditions and comorbidities that should be sought and addressed in the pretransplant evaluation. A comprehensive review of these is not possible in a single article of manageable length; **Boxes 1** and **2** list some of the more important comorbidities and associated conditions for kidney and liver transplant candidates, respectively. Likewise, every transplant candidate should

> **Box 1**
> **Kidney transplant candidates: comorbidities and associated conditions**
>
> Coronary artery disease
>
> Diabetes mellitus
>
> Hypertension
>
> Vascular disease
>
> Cardiorenal syndrome
>
> Anemia
>
> Fluid and electrolyte disturbances

have a routine preanesthetic evaluation as part of his or her workup, including history and pertinent physical examination; that process is not be reexamined here.

KIDNEY TRANSPLANTATION

Kidney transplant improves long-term survival over ongoing dialysis for all patients with end-stage renal disease (ESRD) regardless of cause of failure or demographic

> **Box 2**
> **Liver transplant candidates: comorbidities and associated conditions**
>
> Cardiac
> - Coronary artery disease
> - Cirrhotic cardiomyopathy
>
> Pulmonary/pulmonary vascular
> - Portopulmonary hypertension
> - Hepatopulmonary syndrome
>
> Renal
> - Renal failure
> - Hepatorenal syndrome
> - Hyponatremia
>
> Endocrine
> - Diabetes mellitus
> - Obesity
>
> Hematological
> - Coagulopathy
> - Thrombocytopenia
> - Anemia
>
> Central nervous system
> - Encephalopathy
> - Cerebral edema (in acute failure)
>
> General
> - Sarcopenia

subgrouping, including age.[5] There is, however, an increase in mortality in the immediate posttransplant period continuing out to 3 months post procedure. Cardiovascular disease is the most common cause of death both overall in ESRD and in the immediate posttransplant time frame[6,7]; thus, much effort has gone into identifying the most effective screening and management strategies for cardiovascular disease, and particularly CAD in this population.

CARDIOVASCULAR DISEASE

Cardiovascular disease, and in particular CAD, is highly prevalent in the population with ESRD. Rates of CAD reported in studies of patients undergoing kidney transplant evaluation range from 42% to 81%, with the higher prevalences reported in cohorts with more "high-risk" patients (older, more diabetes) and where a lesser extent of coronary artery stenosis on angiography was considered significant. This high prevalence is unsurprising given that the most common underlying causes of renal failure are diabetes mellitus and hypertension. Also, chronic kidney disease is itself an independent risk factor for cardiovascular disease.[8] The risk of perioperative cardiovascular events in kidney transplant is underscored by the overlap between the predictors in the revised cardiac risk index for perioperative events[9] and conditions common in the patient with ESRD (see **Box 1**).

Identification of CAD

How best to screen for CAD is controversial with several clinical guidelines currently in existence, each with differing recommendations. The differences mainly relate to which patients should go on to further investigations (typically a stress test) to identify CAD. These range from initial stratification based on functional capacity in the American College of Cardiology/American Heart Association (ACC/AHA) guidelines[10] to a recommendation that all transplant candidates should undergo testing from the Kidney Disease Outcomes Quality Initiative (KDOQI) group.[11] Friedman and colleagues[12] retrospectively evaluated 4 different guideline approaches in a cohort of 204 kidney transplant candidates, of whom 17 had been found to have ischemic changes on investigation and 10 underwent pretransplant revascularization. The rate of recommended stress testing varied from 20% using the ACC/AHA guideline to 100% using the KDOQI approach. Although the use of the ACC/AHS guidelines would have resulted in many less stress tests, it would only have identified 4 of the 10 patients who went on to revascularization, indicating that the ACC/AHA guidelines may be too restrictive of further investigation in this population. However, a strategy of testing all candidates may not be an efficient use of resources and comes with the possibility of increased numbers of false-positive results, resulting in further unnecessary investigation. One suggestion is to use stratification schemes incorporating kidney disease–specific factors. In the study described earlier, use of the Lisbon guidelines,[13] which stratify first by presence of diabetes or atherosclerotic disease and then, if absent, by presence of 3 or more kidney disease–specific risk factors (left ventricular hypertrophy [LVH], >1 year on dialysis, age >60 years, dyslipidemia, and hypertension), would have resulted in the identification of all patients who underwent revascularization for the outlay of stress testing in 70% of candidates.[12] This is an improvement on both the most liberal and conservative of regimens, but it is clear that work is still required to optimize screening strategies.

An important point to note in constructing a screening strategy for CAD in patients with ESRD is that symptoms are an unreliable indicator for CAD, with disease being present between 14% and 44% of asymptomatic patients who underwent further evaluation.[14,15] The reason for this is unclear—it may be related to the high prevalence of diabetes mellitus in this population[14]—however, it probably accounts for the poor performance of the ACC/AHA guidelines, which initially stratify based on symptoms, in the study previously discussed.

The issue of which test should be used has been addressed in several studies and has been subjected to a recent systematic review and meta-analysis.[16] The most studied modalities were dobutamine stress echocardiography (DSE, 13 studies) and myocardial perfusion scintography (MPS, 9 studies). Both had moderate sensitivity and specificity in detecting CAD with DSE, demonstrating greater accuracy in the overall evaluation. In addition, DSE was a better discriminator for patients with intermediate risk, leading the investigators to recommend DSE as the screening investigation of choice.

Coronary angiography (CA) remains the gold standard for identifying and quantifying CAD, as well as being necessary when an intervention is planned. The place of CA in the pretransplant evaluation is unclear; in screening algorithms, it is usually reserved for patients who test positive on noninvasive stress testing; however, in published series, it is common to find patients who went directly to CA without prior noninvasive testing or who underwent CA despite a negative noninvasive test. Because a proportion of such patients do have CAD (44% in one study[14]), the reasons such decisions are clinically taken need to be better understood.[17] In addition, there is the concern that CA in the population with ESRD worsens renal function secondary to contrast nephropathy and precipitates the need for dialysis.[18] Historically, CA was deferred until dialysis was initiated; however, this limits investigation and treatment options, particularly for preemptive transplants. This limitation may be less of a concern with modern techniques such as using lower volumes of nonionic contrast, adequate hydration, use of N-acetylcysteine, and careful monitoring. Kumar and colleagues[19] reported no acceleration in decline of renal function after CA. Furthermore, computed tomographic (CT) angiography has been shown to be effective in a population with ESRD[20] and may provide a less invasive means of evaluation.

Other Tests for CAD

Aside from DSE and MPS, several other modalities have been evaluated for identifying CAD in patients with ESRD. Wang and colleagues[16] reviewed the literature, including reports of resting electrocardiography, resting echocardiography, exercise stress testing, coronary calcification evaluation, carotid intimal medial thickness, and digital subtraction fluoroscopy. Less information was available for each (many single studies) than for DSE and MPS, and based on the available evidence, it was believed unlikely that any would prove superior to DSE or MPS.

The role of biomarkers, specifically cardiac troponin T (cTnT) has been investigated. An elevated single measurement of cTnT at the time of evaluation is an independent risk factor for mortality in kidney transplant candidates, both while on the waiting list and posttransplant.[21–24] How this finding should be integrated into pretransplant screening awaits elucidation; an elevated cTnT may identify a risk of mortality independent of the presence of CAD.[24]

Management of CAD

The optimal management for patients identified with stable CAD is currently unclear, with the major area of uncertainty being the place of revascularization, particularly percutaneous intervention (PCI), for identified obstructive lesions. A large randomized study comparing optimal medical therapy with optimal therapy plus revascularization before vascular surgery in patients with obstructive CAD showed no outcome benefit in the revascularization group.[25] A second randomized study again found no benefit to PCI over optimal medial management,[26] with the same result in a reanalysis of the subgroup with chronic kidney disease,[27] although the last 2 studies were not specific to operative candidates. There are no randomized trials specific to kidney transplant patients. Published series have disparate conclusions reporting no revascularization benefit,[28] a benefit only in patients with 3-vessel disease[29] or a survival benefit for revascularization (PCI or coronary artery bypass grafting [CABG]).[14]

Whether periodic cardiac reevaluation is necessary during wait-list time is also unclear; although reevaluation has been recommended,[15] no difference in outcome was found when patients who had periodic reevaluation were compared with those who did not.[30]

A final issue that arises from the cardiovascular evaluation of patients is that the results may lead to an individual not receiving optimal medical care. Patel and colleagues[28] found that the identification of CAD was associated with a failure to list for transplant but was unlikely to lead to a cardiac intervention, thus potentially depriving such individuals of access to potentially survival-enhancing transplant and appropriate cardiovascular therapy. Cardiovascular screening should result in appropriate referral, where indicated, for cardiac disease detected regardless of the effect on transplant candidacy.

Other Cardiac Issues

Patients with chronic kidney disease frequently demonstrate cardiac impairment, a combination referred to as the cardiorenal syndrome. LVH, left ventricular enlargement, and systolic and/or diastolic dysfunction are common, with the most frequent, LVH, being present in nearly three-quarters of patients undergoing dialysis.[31] A low left ventricular ejection fraction (LVEF) is also common with congestive heart failure (CHF) a frequent finding: 30% of patients being initiated on dialysis had CHF, with a further 25% developing it subsequently.[32] In these patients, mortality was twice that of those without CHF.[32] Kidney transplant improves cardiac function. Zolty and colleagues[33] reviewed several prospective studies that showed that cardiac function improves in the posttransplant period, with an increase in LVEF, a decrease in left ventricular size, and a decrease in CHF associated with improved functional status. The longer a patient has been on dialysis before transplant the less likely a return to normal cardiac function posttransplant.[34] Thus, a low ejection fraction or a history of CHF should not be seen as a barrier to transplant. While on the waiting list, patients should have optimal medical management for heart failure; in one study, this only occurred in 25%,[35] although whether optimal management can influence the ongoing decline in cardiac function is unclear.[33]

LIVER TRANSPLANTATION

Patients with ESLD can have significant physiologic alterations associated with their liver failure, which can significantly influence both the expected course and outcome of transplant. The liver transplant procedure is a major abdominal vascular surgery with expected significant cardiovascular stressors occurring during the surgery and the potential for massive blood loss; thus, comorbid conditions that may influence a patient's ability to cope with such insults are important to identify.

SELECTION FOR LIVER TRANSPLANTATION

Most patients presenting for liver transplant evaluation have cirrhotic stage liver disease with consequent complications related to portal hypertension. There are many potential causes, but alcoholic liver disease and chronic hepatitides (particularly hepatitis C) are the most common. There are also several patients who have malignancy not amenable to other treatment but of an extent at which transplant is considered a reasonable option without excessive risk of recurrence. The underlying premises for considering liver transplant are that a patient has liver disease that will not improve with optimal management and that the patient will benefit from undergoing a transplant. When these criteria are met, the question of how to prioritize patients for transplant arises. At present, many countries allocate organs to those patients most likely to die in the shortest time without transplant. Stratification is typically based on the Model for End-stage Liver Disease (MELD) score or one of its variants.[36] The MELD equation uses serum creatinine levels, international normalized ratio, and bilirubin levels and calculates a predicted 3-month mortality. A higher score predicts higher mortality, and patients with higher scores are placed higher on the transplant list. One issue with the use of MELD stratification is that, although it is well validated for the prediction of waiting list mortality, it performs less well as a predictor of posttransplant outcome; patients with the highest MELD scores do have a poorer posttransplant outcome than others, but less than a threshold value discrimination is poor.[37] This drawback has resulted in a search for a more accurate method of outcome prediction; however, to date no well-validated system has been described. In the absence of such a system, the decision to list a patient for transplant is based not solely on MELD but also on evaluation for comorbid conditions known to influence outcome. After the initial evaluation is complete, it is common for a patient to be presented at a selection conference where both the hepatology indication for transplant and the other influencing conditions (medical, psychological, and social) are discussed and the transplant team reaches a consensus decision on candidacy.

Patients with ESLD are at risk for intercurrent critical events either related to their liver failure, such as gastrointestinal bleeding or spontaneous bacterial peritonitis, or other conditions, principally infective. Such patients frequently require intensive care unit (ICU) management for associated shock, coma, and/or respiratory failure.[38] The reported mortality for these patients is 50%.[38] This value raises the question of at what point is a patient so ill that proceeding with liver transplantation is essentially futile or that the mortality risk is at a level at which there is greater overall benefit in giving an available organ to a candidate with better outcome prospects. There are no good data to guide this decision. Many programs consider mechanical ventilation or significant pressor use to be relative contraindications, but such patients have successfully undergone transplants.[39] Ongoing sepsis is usually a contraindication, but at what point in resolving sepsis transplant is advisable is unknown.[40] In the end, most cases are decided on an individual basis after multidisciplinary consultation between the involved medical teams.

ALF is an uncommon condition that accounts for around 5% of liver transplants.[3] Listing for transplant is based on prognosticating nonrecoverability of liver function typically using the King's College criteria.[41]

Although patients with ALF typically do not have the complications associated with cirrhosis and portal hypertension, they can rapidly become critically ill, requiring a high level of ICU support before transplant. Cerebral edema with elevated intracranial pressure (ICP) is a particular concern[42]; if persistently elevated ICP has occurred, evaluation for irreversible brain injury should be undertaken before proceeding with transplantation.

CARDIOVASCULAR DISEASE

Cardiovascular mortality is the leading cause of death in liver transplant recipients, both in the early postoperative period and long term.[43–45] Much of this mortality is related to CAD, resulting in much effort to identify CAD in liver transplant candidates, manage it appropriately, and also determine the risk associated with degrees of CAD.

Coronary Artery Disease

CAD is common in liver transplant candidates, with a prevalence of between 20% and 30%[46,47]; in around 15% of candidates, CAD is unknown at the time of evaluation.[48] The posttransplant outcome of patients with CAD has long been reported to be worse than that of patients without CAD; in the original series addressing this issue, patients with severe CAD had 30% 3-month mortality.[49] After this, screening for CAD was advocated[50] and is now commonplace in US transplant centers. More recently, outcomes for patients with CAD have been reported as improved; in one series, 3-month mortality for both patients with CAD and controls was 2%, although long-term mortality remained higher in the CAD group[51]; in a further multicenter series, no difference in outcome between patients with CAD and without was identified.[52] It is unclear how much this apparent improvement in outcome can be attributed to better management of patients with CAD and how much is to patient selection (ie, exclusion from transplant of patients with more severe CAD); it is, however, interesting to note that the proportion of patients with CAD in many of the published transplant series is less than 5%, much lower than the reported prevalence in patients referred for transplant assessment.[53]

Screening for CAD

The basis for CAD screening in the population with ESLD is noninvasive testing. Pharmacologic stress is most frequently reported as being used with DSE probably the most commonly used method. There have been several series evaluating the performance of DSE in CAD detection and in prediction of pretransplant outcome,[54–61] but interpretation of these studies is confounded by differing selection criteria to identify which patients underwent testing, differing definitions of significant CAD, different outcome measures, and small numbers both overall and of outcome events. Overall, the negative predictive values have been acceptable (75%–100%), but positive predictive values are poor (0%–33%). Similar results are reported for series in which myocardial perfusion imaging was used.[48,62–64] These findings are similar to the effectiveness of stress testing in the noncardiac population in general.[10] These findings suggest that pharmacologic testing may be useful to identify patients at low risk but that further investigation is required to identify CAD in those with a positive study.

At present, at least in US transplant centers, the most widely used approach to initial screening for CAD follows the recommendations from the American Association for the Study of Liver Diseases.[65] These recommendations call for noninvasive testing in patients older than 50 years, with a clinical or family history of heart disease, with diabetes mellitus, and who are chronic smokers. A negative test result is reassuring; positive test result typically leads to further investigation, usually CA.

CA defines the anatomic extent of CAD and is a necessary step if intervention is being considered. Some groups have advocated proceeding directly to CA in patients deemed to be at high risk for CAD[62,66]; however, how to identify these individuals is not well defined. Guidelines for cardiovascular risk evaluation in noncardiac surgery do not support this position.[10,67]

Performing CA in patients with ESLD raises some concerns, most notably of periprocedural bleeding and of worsening renal function. A case control study reported that patients with ESLD required more blood and blood products and had a higher incidence of postprocedure pseudoaneurysm but overall concluded that CA can be safely accomplished with appropriate attention to coagulation.[68] CT angiography may also be useful in decreasing morbidity in this population. The issue of CA and renal function is discussed earlier, in the kidney transplant section.

Troponin

Pretransplant elevation of troponin levels has been reported as a strong predictor of both posttransplant cardiovascular events and overall mortality in liver transplant patients.[69,70] How this information can be used in the preoperative stratification and management of these patients is currently unclear.

Management of CAD

There is a paucity of evidence regarding how to manage CAD in the liver transplant candidate. Although randomized studies have suggested no benefit to revascularization over optimal medical management in the population with CAD in general and in elective vascular surgery patients,[25,26] the practice most pursued in liver transplant programs is to correct significant lesions, with PCI being the most frequent strategy. Bare metal stents are usually deployed because of the shorter (1 month) recommendation for dual antiplatelet therapy.[71] CABG is infrequently advocated as the risk of acute hepatic decompensation in the perioperative period, the risk being high for patients with ESLD[72]; however, there are reports of successful combined liver transplant and CABG.[73]

The severity of cardiac disease at which liver transplant is considered too high risk to be an appropriate procedure is not defined; however, severity of CAD and its consequences are one of the considerations in patient selection. Situations in which denial of transplant are considered include the patient with noncorrectable disease (for example diffuse disease) and easily inducible ischemia, patients with low resting ejection fraction, and patients with marginal resting cardiac performance who demonstrate no improvement or worsening with stress.

Exercise Testing

Exercise testing for pretransplant evaluation has been infrequently performed, most likely because of the high proportion of patients with ESLD with severe exercise limitation.[74] There has been interest in using cardiopulmonary exercise testing (CPET) for pretransplant evaluation, particularly using values derived from submaximal testing. Prentis and colleagues[75] reported that 90% of a series of patients with ESLD could exercise adequately for this purpose and that stratification by anaerobic threshold was highly predictive of 90-day posttransplant mortality. This finding is of interest, as CPET identifies more than the existence of a specific condition—as evaluation for CAD does—and provides a quantification of functional capacity and reserve which is conceptually appealing in assessing suitability for a major procedure. What the true significance of this finding is awaits further elucidation.

OTHER CARDIAC CONSIDERATIONS
Valvular Disease

There are no good outcome data to guide the selection and management of liver transplant candidates with valvular dysfunction; thus, practice must be guided by an understanding of both the valvular and cardiac functions of the candidate and the anticipated hemodynamic stresses associated with transplant. Those with severe valvular dysfunction are typically not considered transplant candidates without correction of the valvular lesion, if this is feasible. Mild valvular lesions are not a barrier. Intermediate cases should be approached on an individualized basis.

Left Ventricular Outflow Tract Obstruction

Dynamic left ventricular outflow tract obstruction may be detected on DSE during pretransplant evaluation. Patients with ESLD may be at increased risk for this given their typical hemodynamic profile of a high cardiac output and low peripheral resistance. Such patients have successfully undergone transplant with appropriate intraoperative management.[76,77]

Patients with hypertrophic cardiomyopathy have also successfully undergone transplant, some after alcohol septal ablation[78]; however, there is no guidance on when pretransplant intervention should be performed.

Cirrhotic Cardiomyopathy

A cirrhotic cardiomyopathy (CCM) has been characterized in patients with ESLD. It consists of systolic dysfunction, in particular impaired response to stress, diastolic dysfunction, and electrophysiologic abnormalities evidenced by a prolonged QT interval,[79] changes that improve posttransplant.[80] The influence of CCM on transplant outcome is unclear; the prevalence of diastolic dysfunction has recently been reported as 67% in patients with ESLD; it did not have a significant independent effect on survival.[81]

PULMONARY AND PULMONARY VASCULAR DISEASE

Alterations in pulmonary mechanics and gas exchange are common in ESLD. An increased alveolar-arterial gradient has been reported in 40%.[82] In many cases, this is secondary to restrictive changes resulting from ascites, pleural effusion, and obesity[83]; however, some patients have one of the specific liver failure–related syndromes, HPS and portopulmonary hypertension (POPH), which can influence transplant candidacy and outcome.

Hepatopulmonary Syndrome

HPS is characterized by a defect in oxygenation associated with pulmonary vascular dilation and a consequent intrapulmonary shunt. Patients are often dyspneic, have clubbing, and may exhibit orthodeoxia and platypnea, but there are no diagnostic signs or symptoms.[84] Diagnosis is made by demonstrating a pulmonary shunt either by contrast echocardiography (showing delayed contrast appearance after 3–6 cardiac cycles in the left side of the heart) or by radiolabeled albumin macroaggregate scanning, which allows the shunt to be quantified.[85] Some degree of pulmonary shunting may be present in almost 50% of transplant candidates.[86] Severity is categorized from mild to very severe by the arterial P_{O_2} on room air; very severe cases have a P_{O_2} less than 50 mm Hg. Patients with ESLD and HPS have an inferior survival to those without,[87] and currently in the United States, patients with HPS gain an enhanced status on the waiting list. Previously, patients with very severe HPS were reported as having a high posttransplant mortality[88]; however, more recently, improved outcomes in this group have been reported,[89] such that severe HPS should not be considered a contraindication to transplant. Posttransplant hypoxemia resolves, but this can take more than 12 months.[89]

Portopulmonary Hypertension

POPH is pulmonary hypertension (a mean pulmonary artery pressure [MPAP] ≥25 mm Hg) in association with portal hypertension with no other identifiable cause for pulmonary hypertension.[90] It is uncommon in ESLD, occurring in approximately 6% of liver transplant candidates.[91] It is classified into mild, moderate, and severe, based on measured MPAP (25–35, 35–45, and >45 mm Hg, respectively).[85] The importance of this is that mild POPH is associated with excellent outcome after liver transplantation, whereas moderate to severe POPH is associated with high perioperative mortality, greater than 50% if PAP is greater than 35 mm Hg and pulmonary vascular resistance (PVR) is greater than 250 dyn·s·cm^{-5}.[85,92]

Patients with POPH often have no specific symptoms; therefore, screening for POPH should be part of the pretransplant evaluation for all candidates. The most used screening test is resting echocardiography, with estimation of right ventricular (RV) (hence pulmonary artery [PA]) systolic pressure by Doppler assessment of the tricuspid regurgitant jet. Patients identified as having high PA pressure, typically an estimated RV systolic greater than 50 mm Hg, should then proceed to catheterization of the right side of the heart to measure both actual PA pressures and evaluate hemodynamics.[85] Catheterization confirmation is necessary, as 35% of those with elevated RV systolic pressure on Doppler have been found to have either acceptable PA pressures on catheterization or to have identifiable causes for the high PA pressure, such as volume overload.[93]

Patients identified with moderate to severe pulmonary hypertension (MPAP >35 mm Hg and PVR >250 dyn·s·cm^{-5}) should have transplant deferred and medical therapy for pulmonary hypertension initiated; transplant can then be considered if and when pulmonary hemodynamics have improved to within the acceptable range.[65]

OTHER ORGANS

Most pancreas transplants are in concert with kidney transplants; the pretransplant evaluation is similar to that described for kidney. There is little published information specific to the evaluation of patient for intestinal or multivisceral transplant.

REFERENCES

1. Global observatory on donation and transplantation. 2013. Available at: http://www.transplant-observatory.org/Pages/home.aspx. Accessed February 21, 2013.
2. Health Resources and Services Administration (HRSA), Department of Health and Human Services (HHS). Organ procurement and transplantation network. Final rule. Fed Regist 2013;78:40033–42. Available at: http://optn.transplant.hrsa.gov/data/. Accessed February 21, 2013.
3. 2011 Annual Report of the U.S. Organ procurement and transplantation network and the scientific registry of transplant recipients. Rockville (MD): Department of Health and Human Services HRaSA, Healthcare Systems Bureau, Division of Transplantation; 2012.
4. United Network for Organ Sharing. UNOS Bylaws Organ Procurement and Transplantation Network Bylaws Appendix B Attachment I -XIII. 2011. Available at: http://optn.transplant.hrsa.gov/policiesAndBylaws/bylaws.asp. Accessed September 17, 2013.
5. Wolfe RA, Ashby VB, Milford EL, et al. Comparison of mortality in all patients on dialysis, patients on dialysis awaiting transplantation, and recipients of a first cadaveric transplant. N Engl J Med 1999;341:1725–30.
6. Aalten J, Hoogeveen EK, Roodnat JI, et al. Associations between pre-kidney-transplant risk factors and post-transplant cardiovascular events and death. Transpl Int 2008;21:985–91.

7. Lentine KL, Hurst FP, Jindal RM, et al. Cardiovascular risk assessment among potential kidney transplant candidates: approaches and controversies. Am J Kidney Dis 2010;55:152–67.

8. Tonelli M, Wiebe N, Culleton B, et al. Chronic kidney disease and mortality risk: a systematic review. J Am Soc Nephrol 2006;17:2034–47.

9. Lee TH, Marcantonio ER, Mangione CM, et al. Derivation and prospective validation of a simple index for prediction of cardiac risk of major noncardiac surgery. Circulation 1999;100:1043–9.

10. Fleisher LA, Beckman JA, Brown KA, et al. ACC/AHA 2007 guidelines on perioperative cardiovascular evaluation and care for noncardiac surgery: executive summary: a report of the American College of Cardiology/American Heart Association Task Force on Practice Guidelines (Writing Committee to Revise the 2002 Guidelines on Perioperative Cardiovascular Evaluation for Noncardiac Surgery) Developed in Collaboration With the American Society of Echocardiography, American Society of Nuclear Cardiology, Heart Rhythm Society, Society of Cardiovascular Anesthesiologists, Society for Cardiovascular Angiography and Interventions, Society for Vascular Medicine and Biology, and Society for Vascular Surgery. J Am Coll Cardiol 2007;50:1707–32.

11. K/DOQI Workgroup. K/DOQI clinical practice guidelines for cardiovascular disease in dialysis patients. Am J Kidney Dis 2005;45:S1–153.

12. Friedman SE, Palac RT, Zlotnick DM, et al. A call to action: variability in guidelines for cardiac evaluation before renal transplantation. Clin J Am Soc Nephrol 2011;6:1185–91.

13. Abbud-Filho M, Adams PL, Alberu J, et al. A report of the Lisbon Conference on the care of the kidney transplant recipient. Transplantation 2007;83:S1–22.

14. Kahn MR, Fallahi A, Kim MC, et al. Coronary artery disease in a large renal transplant population: implications for management. Am J Transplant 2011;11: 2665–74.

15. Leonardi G, Tamagnone M, Ferro M, et al. Assessment of cardiovascular risk in waiting-listed renal transplant patients: a single center experience in 558 cases. Clin Transplant 2009;23:653–9.

16. Wang LW, Fahim MA, Hayen A, et al. Cardiac testing for coronary artery disease in potential kidney transplant recipients. Cochrane Database Syst Rev 2011;(12): CD008691.

17. Kittleson MM. Preoperative cardiac evaluation of kidney transplant recipients: does testing matter? Am J Transplant 2011;11:2553–4.

18. Mehran R, Aymong ED, Nikolsky E, et al. A simple risk score for prediction of contrast-induced nephropathy after percutaneous coronary intervention: development and initial validation. J Am Coll Cardiol 2004;44:1393–9.

19. Kumar N, Dahri L, Brown W, et al. Effect of elective coronary angiography on glomerular filtration rate in patients with advanced chronic kidney disease. Clin J Am Soc Nephrol 2009;4:1907–13.

20. de Bie MK, Buiten MS, Gaasbeek A, et al. CT coronary angiography is feasible for the assessment of coronary artery disease in chronic dialysis patients, despite high average calcium scores. PLoS One 2013;8:e67936.

21. Connolly GM, Cunningham R, McNamee PT, et al. Troponin T is an independent predictor of mortality in renal transplant recipients. Nephrol Dial Transplant 2008;23:1019–25.

22. Hickson LJ, Cosio FG, El-Zoghby ZM, et al. Survival of patients on the kidney transplant wait list: relationship to cardiac troponin T. Am J Transplant 2008;8: 2352–9.

23. Hickson LT, El-Zoghby ZM, Lorenz EC, et al. Patient survival after kidney transplantation: relationship to pretransplant cardiac troponin T levels. Am J Transplant 2009;9:1354–61.
24. Sharma R, Gaze DC, Pellerin D, et al. Ischemia-modified albumin predicts mortality in ESRD. Am J Kidney Dis 2006;47:493–502.
25. McFalls EO, Ward HB, Moritz TE, et al. Coronary-artery revascularization before elective major vascular surgery. N Engl J Med 2004;351:2795–804.
26. Boden WE, O'Rourke RA, Teo KK, et al. Optimal medical therapy with or without PCI for stable coronary disease. N Engl J Med 2007;356:1503–16.
27. Sedlis SP, Jurkovitz CT, Hartigan PM, et al. Optimal medical therapy with or without percutaneous coronary intervention for patients with stable coronary artery disease and chronic kidney disease. Am J Cardiol 2009;104:1647–53.
28. Patel RK, Mark PB, Johnston N, et al. Prognostic value of cardiovascular screening in potential renal transplant recipients: a single-center prospective observational study. Am J Transplant 2008;8:1673–83.
29. Hage FG, Smalheiser S, Zoghbi GJ, et al. Predictors of survival in patients with end-stage renal disease evaluated for kidney transplantation. Am J Cardiol 2007;100:1020–5.
30. Gill JS, Ma I, Landsberg D, et al. Cardiovascular events and investigation in patients who are awaiting cadaveric kidney transplantation. J Am Soc Nephrol 2005;16:808–16.
31. Foley RN, Parfrey PS, Harnett JD, et al. Clinical and echocardiographic disease in patients starting end-stage renal disease therapy. Kidney Int 1995;47:186–92.
32. Harnett JD, Foley RN, Kent GM, et al. Congestive heart failure in dialysis patients: prevalence, incidence, prognosis and risk factors. Kidney Int 1995;47:884–90.
33. Zolty R, Hynes PJ, Vittorio TJ. Severe left ventricular systolic dysfunction may reverse with renal transplantation: uremic cardiomyopathy and cardiorenal syndrome. Am J Transplant 2008;8:2219–24.
34. Wali RK, Wang GS, Gottlieb SS, et al. Effect of kidney transplantation on left ventricular systolic dysfunction and congestive heart failure in patients with end-stage renal disease. J Am Coll Cardiol 2005;45:1051–60.
35. Trespalacios FC, Taylor AJ, Agodoa LY, et al. Heart failure as a cause for hospitalization in chronic dialysis patients. Am J Kidney Dis 2003;41:1267–77.
36. Kamath PS, Wiesner RH, Malinchoc M, et al. A model to predict survival in patients with end-stage liver disease. Hepatology 2001;33:464–70.
37. Jacob M, Copley LP, Lewsey JD, et al. Pretransplant MELD score and post liver transplantation survival in the UK and Ireland. Liver Transpl 2004;10:903–7.
38. Das V, Boelle PY, Galbois A, et al. Cirrhotic patients in the medical intensive care unit: early prognosis and long-term survival. Crit Care Med 2010;38:2108–16.
39. Brown RS Jr, Kumar KS, Russo MW, et al. Model for end-stage liver disease and Child-Turcotte-Pugh score as predictors of pretransplantation disease severity, posttransplantation outcome, and resource utilization in United Network for Organ Sharing status 2A patients. Liver Transpl 2002;8:278–84.
40. Findlay JY, Fix OK, Paugam-Burtz C, et al. Critical care of the end-stage liver disease patient awaiting liver transplantation. Liver Transpl 2011;17:496–510.
41. O'Grady JG, Alexander GJ, Hayllar KM, et al. Early indicators of prognosis in fulminant hepatic failure. Gastroenterology 1989;97:439–45.
42. Wijdicks EF, Plevak DJ, Rakela J, et al. Clinical and radiologic features of cerebral edema in fulminant hepatic failure. Mayo Clin Proc 1995;70:119–24.

43. Fouad TR, Abdel-Razek WM, Burak KW, et al. Prediction of cardiac complications after liver transplantation. Transplantation 2009;87:763–70.
44. Johnston SD, Morris JK, Cramb R, et al. Cardiovascular morbidity and mortality after orthotopic liver transplantation. Transplantation 2002;73:901–6.
45. Pruthi J, Medkiff KA, Esrason KT, et al. Analysis of causes of death in liver transplant recipients who survived more than 3 years. Liver Transpl 2001;7: 811–5.
46. Carey WD, Dumot JA, Pimentel RR, et al. The prevalence of coronary artery disease in liver transplant candidates over age 50. Transplantation 1995;59: 859–64.
47. Kalaitzakis E, Rosengren A, Skommevik T, et al. Coronary artery disease in patients with liver cirrhosis. Dig Dis Sci 2010;55:467–75.
48. Aydinalp A, Bal U, Atar I, et al. Value of stress myocardial perfusion scanning in diagnosis of severe coronary artery disease in liver transplantation candidates. Transplant Proc 2009;41:3757–60.
49. Plotkin JS, Scott VL, Pinna A, et al. Morbidity and mortality in patients with coronary artery disease undergoing orthotopic liver transplantation. Liver Transpl Surg 1996;2:426–30.
50. Plevak DJ. Stress echocardiography identifies coronary artery disease in liver transplant candidates. Liver Transpl Surg 1998;4:337–9.
51. Diedrich DA, Findlay JY, Harrison BA, et al. Influence of coronary artery disease on outcomes after liver transplantation. Transplant Proc 2008;40: 3554–7.
52. Wray C, Scovotti JC, Tobis J, et al. Liver transplantation outcome in patients with angiographically proven coronary artery disease: a multi-institutional study. Am J Transplant 2013;13:184–91.
53. Findlay JY. Coronary artery disease and liver transplantation. In: Milan Z, editor. Cardiovascular disease and liver transplantation. New York: Nova Science Publishers; 2011. p. 31–48.
54. Donovan CL, Marcovitz PA, Punch JD, et al. Two-dimensional and dobutamine stress echocardiography in the preoperative assessment of patients with end-stage liver disease prior to orthotopic liver transplantation. Transplantation 1996;61:1180–8.
55. Findlay JY, Keegan MT, Pellikka PP, et al. Preoperative dobutamine stress echocardiography, intraoperative events, and intraoperative myocardial injury in liver transplantation. Transplant Proc 2005;37:2209–13.
56. Harinstein ME, Flaherty JD, Ansari AH, et al. Predictive value of dobutamine stress echocardiography for coronary artery disease detection in liver transplant candidates. Am J Transplant 2008;8:1523–8.
57. Plotkin JS, Benitez RM, Kuo PC, et al. Dobutamine stress echocardiography for preoperative cardiac risk stratification in patients undergoing orthotopic liver transplantation. Liver Transpl Surg 1998;4:253–7.
58. Safadi A, Homsi M, Maskoun W, et al. Perioperative risk predictors of cardiac outcomes in patients undergoing liver transplantation surgery. Circulation 2009;120:1189–94.
59. Tsutsui JM, Mukherjee S, Elhendy A, et al. Value of dobutamine stress myocardial contrast perfusion echocardiography in patients with advanced liver disease. Liver Transpl 2006;12:592–9.
60. Umphrey LG, Hurst RT, Eleid MF, et al. Preoperative dobutamine stress echocardiographic findings and subsequent short-term adverse cardiac events after orthotopic liver transplantation. Liver Transpl 2008;14:886–92.

61. Williams K, Lewis JF, Davis G, et al. Dobutamine stress echocardiography in patients undergoing liver transplantation evaluation. Transplantation 2000;69: 2354–6.
62. Davidson CJ, Gheorghiade M, Flaherty JD, et al. Predictive value of stress myocardial perfusion imaging in liver transplant candidates. Am J Cardiol 2002;89:359–60.
63. Kryzhanovski VA, Beller GA. Usefulness of preoperative noninvasive radionuclide testing for detecting coronary artery disease in candidates for liver transplantation. Am J Cardiol 1997;79:986–8.
64. Zoghbi GJ, Patel AD, Ershadi RE, et al. Usefulness of preoperative stress perfusion imaging in predicting prognosis after liver transplantation. Am J Cardiol 2003;92:1066–71.
65. Murray KF, Carithers RL Jr. AASLD practice guidelines: evaluation of the patient for liver transplantation. Hepatology 2005;41:1407–32.
66. Raval Z, Harinstein ME, Skaro AI, et al. Cardiovascular risk assessment of the liver transplant candidate. J Am Coll Cardiol 2011;58:223–31.
67. Poldermans D, Bax JJ, Boersma E, et al. Guidelines for pre-operative cardiac risk assessment and perioperative cardiac management in non-cardiac surgery: the Task Force for Preoperative Cardiac Risk Assessment and Perioperative Cardiac Management in Non-cardiac Surgery of the European Society of Cardiology (ESC) and endorsed by the European Society of Anaesthesiology (ESA). Eur Heart J 2009;30:2769–812.
68. Sharma M, Yong C, Majure D, et al. Safety of cardiac catheterization in patients with end-stage liver disease awaiting liver transplantation. Am J Cardiol 2009; 103:742–6.
69. Coss E, Watt KD, Pedersen R, et al. Predictors of cardiovascular events after liver transplantation: a role for pretransplant serum troponin levels. Liver Transpl 2011;17:23–31.
70. Watt KD, Coss E, Pedersen RA, et al. Pretransplant serum troponin levels are highly predictive of patient and graft survival following liver transplantation. Liver Transpl 2010;16:990–8.
71. Grines CL, Bonow RO, Casey DE Jr, et al. Prevention of premature discontinuation of dual antiplatelet therapy in patients with coronary artery stents: a science advisory from the American Heart Association, American College of Cardiology, Society for Cardiovascular Angiography and Interventions, American College of Surgeons, and American Dental Association, with representation from the American College of Physicians. J Am Coll Cardiol 2007; 49:734–9.
72. Filsoufi F, Salzberg SP, Rahmanian PB, et al. Early and late outcome of cardiac surgery in patients with liver cirrhosis. Liver Transpl 2007;13:990–5.
73. DeStephano CC, Harrison BA, Mordecai M, et al. Anesthesia for combined cardiac surgery and liver transplant. J Cardiothorac Vasc Anesth 2010;24: 285–92.
74. Dharancy S, Lemyze M, Boleslawski E, et al. Impact of impaired aerobic capacity on liver transplant candidates. Transplantation 2008;86:1077–83.
75. Prentis JM, Manas DM, Trenell MI, et al. Submaximal cardiopulmonary exercise testing predicts 90-day survival after liver transplantation. Liver Transpl 2012;18: 152–9.
76. Lee AR, Kim YR, Ham JS, et al. Dynamic left ventricular outflow tract obstruction in living donor liver transplantation recipients - a report of two cases. Korean J Anesthesiol 2010;59(Suppl):S128–32.

77. Roy D, Ralley FE. Anesthetic management of a patient with dynamic left ventricular outflow tract obstruction with systolic anterior movement of the mitral valve undergoing redo-orthotopic liver transplantation. J Cardiothorac Vasc Anesth 2012;26:274–6.

78. Hage FG, Bravo PE, Zoghbi GJ, et al. Hypertrophic obstructive cardiomyopathy in liver transplant patients. Cardiol J 2008;15:74–9.

79. Moller S, Henriksen JH. Cirrhotic cardiomyopathy. J Hepatol 2010;53:179–90.

80. Torregrosa M, Aguade S, Dos L, et al. Cardiac alterations in cirrhosis: reversibility after liver transplantation. J Hepatol 2005;42:68–74.

81. Alexopoulou A, Papatheodoridis G, Pouriki S, et al. Diastolic myocardial dysfunction does not affect survival in patients with cirrhosis. Transpl Int 2012;25:1174–81.

82. Przybylowski T, Krenke R, Fangrat A, et al. Gas exchange abnormalities in patients listed for liver transplantation. J Physiol Pharmacol 2006;57(Suppl 4):313–23.

83. Yao EH, Kong BC, Hsue GL, et al. Pulmonary function changes in cirrhosis of the liver. Am J Gastroenterol 1987;82:352–4.

84. Rodriguez-Roisin R, Krowka MJ. Hepatopulmonary syndrome–a liver-induced lung vascular disorder. N Engl J Med 2008;358:2378–87.

85. Rodriguez-Roisin R, Krowka MJ, Herve P, et al. Pulmonary-hepatic vascular disorders (PHD). Eur Respir J 2004;24:861–80.

86. Agarwal PD, Hughes PJ, Runo JR, et al. The clinical significance of intrapulmonary vascular dilations in liver transplant candidates. Clin Transplant 2013;27:148–53.

87. Schiffer E, Majno P, Mentha G, et al. Hepatopulmonary syndrome increases the postoperative mortality rate following liver transplantation: a prospective study in 90 patients. Am J Transplant 2006;6:1430–7.

88. Arguedas MR, Abrams GA, Krowka MJ, et al. Prospective evaluation of outcomes and predictors of mortality in patients with hepatopulmonary syndrome undergoing liver transplantation. Hepatology 2003;37:192–7.

89. Gupta S, Castel H, Rao RV, et al. Improved survival after liver transplantation in patients with hepatopulmonary syndrome. Am J Transplant 2010;10:354–63.

90. Galie N, Hoeper MM, Humbert M, et al. Guidelines for the diagnosis and treatment of pulmonary hypertension: the Task Force for the Diagnosis and Treatment of Pulmonary Hypertension of the European Society of Cardiology (ESC) and the European Respiratory Society (ERS), endorsed by the International Society of Heart and Lung Transplantation (ISHLT). Eur Heart J 2009;30:2493–537.

91. Colle IO, Moreau R, Godinho E, et al. Diagnosis of portopulmonary hypertension in candidates for liver transplantation: a prospective study. Hepatology 2003;37:401–9.

92. Krowka MJ, Plevak DJ, Findlay JY, et al. Pulmonary hemodynamics and perioperative cardiopulmonary-related mortality in patients with portopulmonary hypertension undergoing liver transplantation. Liver Transpl 2000;6:443–50.

93. Krowka MJ, Swanson KL, Frantz RP, et al. Portopulmonary hypertension: results from a 10-year screening algorithm. Hepatology 2006;44:1502–10.

Intraoperative Care of the Transplant Patient

Michael D. Spiro, MD, Helge Eilers, MD*

KEYWORDS

- Transplantation • Anesthetic management • Liver • Kidney • Pancreas
- Comorbidities

KEY POINTS

- Patients presenting for abdominal organ transplantation often have significant comorbidities, including cardiovascular and pulmonary disease, posing numerous challenges to the anesthesiologist in the perioperative period.
- Intraoperative management for abdominal organ transplantation is highly variable between transplant centers and depends on factors such as experience of surgical and anesthesia teams as well as available resources.
- Abdominal organ transplantations are major surgeries involving multiple vascular anastomoses. Patients may have advanced disease at the time of surgery, increasing the risk for morbidity and mortality.
- Adequate preparation including preoperative workup and risk stratification, planning of vascular access, blood product management, and preparation for possible complications is important to minimize the risk of perioperative morbidity and mortality. Standardization of protocols within a transplant center is important in that aspect.
- In this article we try to provide background and practical information helpful in establishing or improving protocols for intraoperative management. However, the management will have to be adapted to the practices of each particular transplant center and established protocols cannot simply be transferred to a new setting.

RENAL TRANSPLANTATION
Brief Overview

Patients presenting for renal transplant have extensive comorbidities, most importantly cardiovascular disease, posing numerous challenges to the anesthetist in the perioperative period. Organs from living donors confer the best short- and long-term outcomes.[1] The 3-year graft survival is 88% with cadaveric organs and 93% from living organ donation.[2]

Anesthesia and Perioperative Care, University of California San Francisco School of Medicine, 513 Parnassus Avenue, Room S-436, Box 0427, San Francisco, CA 94143, USA
* Corresponding author.
E-mail address: EilersH@anesthesia.ucsf.edu

Anesthesiology Clin 31 (2013) 705–721
http://dx.doi.org/10.1016/j.anclin.2013.09.005
1932-2275/13/$ – see front matter © 2013 Elsevier Inc. All rights reserved.

Transplant Recipient—Anesthetic Management

Transplant recipients undergo extensive preoperative workup to optimize the intraoperative course. However, waiting times for transplant can be extremely long and a thorough preoperative review is necessary. In addition, the fluid status should be assessed in detail. Patients would frequently have undergone recent dialysis and may be significantly fluid depleted resulting in potential cardiovascular instability after induction of anesthesia. If dialysis has been recently performed, residual effects of anticoagulants can be problematic. Patients often know that their "dry weight" and current weight on the day of surgery may aid assessment. Recently drawn laboratory test results are also required with particular attention to the serum potassium level, which is frequently high in end-stage renal failure. Potassium levels greater than 6 mmol/L may warrant a delay in surgery while this is corrected.[3] Patients are also expected to be relatively anemic secondary to chronic kidney disease despite many having erythropoietin supplementation.

Coagulation studies (prothrombin time and partial thromboplastin time) are routinely performed before surgery. Uremia causes platelet dysfunction, and therefore hemostatic clot formation can be hindered (prolonged bleeding time). This effect may also be secondary to the effects of anemia in end-stage renal failure; correction of anemia to packed cell volume greater than 30% reduces the bleeding risk dramatically.[4]

A medication history should be taken, with particular attention to antihypertensive drugs. Evidence suggests that β-blockade should be continued in the perioperative period[5,6] to reduce the risk of myocardial infarction, although no rigorous studies have been conducted in the kidney transplant population. Consideration should be given to withholding angiotensin-converting-enzyme inhibitor (ACE-I) and angiotensin II receptor blocker (A2RBs) on the day of surgery because of the risk of severe and refractory hypotension postinduction.[7]

Anesthetic Choice

The initial renal transplants were performed exclusively under spinal anesthesia, and there are recent reports of centers using regional techniques with good outcomes.[8–11] More commonly, however, endotracheal intubation is performed and anesthesia is maintained with volatile anesthetics, although total IV anesthetic techniques have also been shown to be effective and safe.[12] When maintenance with volatile anesthetic has been compared with total intravenous anesthesia (TIVA) techniques, no difference in outcome has been shown.[13] Concerns exist around the use of sevoflurane because of its metabolism to potentially nephrotoxic fluoride ions and the production of Compound A in a reaction with sodium or barium hydroxide lime. No study has shown a clinically relevant risk to renal function regardless of fresh gas flow rates, even in patients with preexisting renal insufficiency.[14,15] However, controlled studies have not been performed in patients undergoing renal transplant.

Monitoring

Depending on the patient's comorbidities, renal transplantation may be performed with standard American Society of Anesthesiologists (ASA) monitoring alone. Invasive monitoring is institution and patient specific and not always routine. Central line insertion is reserved for patients with specific indications, such as poor peripheral IV access or need for monitoring of cardiac filling pressures. No benefit has been shown in graft function by targeting a specific central venous pressure (CVP) or fluid management based on venous pressure.[16] If venous pressure measurement is required, peripheral venous pressures (transduced via a peripheral IV) have been shown to have a tight correlation to CVP without the need for central venous access.[17]

Similarly, arterial line insertion is only truly indicated in patients who are anticipated to have significant cardiovascular instability under general anesthesia, for example, those with severe coronary artery disease (CAD), uncontrolled hypertension, poor cardiac function, or significant valvular lesions. In these patients, it may be prudent to site the arterial line awake, before induction. Severe cardiac arrhythmias are rare in this patient population.[18]

Vascular Access

Patients may have had multiple fistulae for dialysis and recurrent hospital admissions with attempts at IV access. Consequently, these patients may present significant challenges when attempting to obtain IV access. A well-functioning 20-gauge IV is usually adequate for induction with a second, larger IV sited under anesthesia.

Induction

Patients with uremia and other risk factors, such as gastroparesis secondary to diabetes, are at high risk of gastric aspiration. A rapid sequence induction (RSI) with cricoid pressure should be considered along with sodium citrate pretreatment to increase gastric pH, thereby reducing pulmonary damage should aspiration occur. RSI can be performed with caution using rocuronium or suxamethonium. Rocuronium can be anticipated to give a prolonged block because of the reduced renal elimination (49 minutes for 25% first twitch (T1) recovery vs 32 minutes in patients with normal renal function), although predominant hepatic metabolism occurs allowing for safe use at induction.[19,20] Suxamethonium will cause an increase in plasma potassium levels to a similar extent (0.5 mmol/L) to that seen in the general population.[3] This drug can be used safely as long as the preoperative potassium level is below 5 mmol/L.[3] About 20% of patients with end-stage renal failure (ESRF) have been shown to have below normal plasma cholinesterase activity. Prolonged neuromuscular blockade is only seen to occur in patients with an atypical form of plasma cholinesterase.[21]

Hypnosis is usually induced with a judicious dose of propofol. In studies, patients with end-stage renal failure have been shown to require significantly more propofol to achieve hypnosis and target bispectral index (BIS) values than healthy controls, probably because of a hyperdynamic circulation and increased intravascular volume and hence volume of distribution.[22] However, cautious induction dosing remains advisable in these patients because of their cardiovascular comorbidities. Maintenance of muscle relaxation should be provided with nonrenally excreted drugs such as atracurium or cisatracurium, which rely predominantly on Hofmann degradation.

In some institutions, the pressor response to intubation is attenuated with esmolol, 0.5 to 1 mg/kg, rather than high-dose opioids to minimize postinduction hypotension. Once fascia is dissected, the surgery is relatively unstimulating, and titrating a short-acting cardioselective β-blocker allows for precise heart rate control and maintenance of adequate diastolic pressure in patients at high risk of myocardial ischemia. Opioid analgesia is often titrated toward the end of surgery, which aids in the maintenance of adequate perfusion pressures throughout the procedure without the need for exogenous vasopressors, which may contribute to reduced renal blood flow and graft vasoconstriction. Fentanyl is typically used because of its limited renal elimination (7%) and is therefore less likely to accumulate.

After induction, meticulous attention to positioning of the patient is required and, in particular, to protecting arteriovenous (AV) fistulae. AV fistulae should also be monitored periodically throughout surgery. Perioperative loss of fistula function can be problematic because a proportion of patients have delayed graft function and require dialysis postoperatively.

Immunosuppressive medications to prevent graft rejection are administered by the anesthesiologist intraoperatively and should be discussed with the surgical team. Methylprednisolone is often given and may modulate the patient's pain response and hence analgesic requirements postoperatively.

Fluid Management

Controversies exist regarding the appropriate volume and constitution of IV fluid administered during renal transplantation. As discussed earlier, these patients are often fluid deplete on arrival to the operating room because of recent dialysis and preoperative starvation. Adequate fluid loading is required to improve immediate graft function and prevent intraoperative hypotension. A blood volume of 70 mL/kg has been shown to correlate with immediate graft function in living related renal transplantation.[23]

When a CVP line is inserted, targeting a CVP of 10 to 15 mm Hg has been advocated to optimize cardiac output and renal perfusion.

Concerns regarding hyperkalemia have led to the widespread administration of potassium-deplete fluid, for example, 0.9% saline. Recent surveys show that this is the practice during transplantation in 90% of cases in 49 centers across the United States.[24] However, O'Malley and colleagues[25] demonstrated that hyperkalemia (>6.0 mmol/L) and metabolic acidosis were significantly increased in patients undergoing renal transplant who received saline rather than Ringer lactate. Intraoperative albumin administration has been shown to be beneficial for graft function in a dose-dependent manner, presumably because of effective intravascular volume expansion optimizing graft perfusion and minimizing tissue hypoxia.[23]

Blood transfusion in renal transplantation is rare; however, it is prudent to have the recipient's blood typed and screened.

Hemodynamic Management

Intraoperative hypotension can be minimized via adequate fluid administration and judicious use of induction agents and opioids. Reperfusion injury may occur on unclamping of the iliac vessels and perfusion of the graft.

Potent vasoconstrictors with α-adrenergic activity, such as phenylephrine, should be avoided during renal transplantation because of concerns regarding vasoconstriction in the graft and should only be used as a last resort. Vessels within the transplanted organ are more sensitive to vasoconstriction than the systemic arterioles, hence blood flow in the graft could become compromised.[26] Dopamine infusion can be used as an inotropic agent to improve mean arterial pressure if hypotension becomes problematic.

Discussion of Adjuvant Drugs

In addition to ensuring adequate perfusion of the kidney with fluid loading, osmotic and loop diuretics are frequently administered to enhance urine output. A recent survey demonstrated extensive variation in intraoperative diuretic use between different transplant centers, and an evidence base for their use remains controversial.[27]

Typically, furosemide and mannitol are used to promote diuresis and dopamine is infused to enhance renal blood flow in an attempt to optimize graft function.

Mannitol is freely filtered at the nephron and exerts an osmotic effect increasing urine volume. Mannitol may protect the renal tubules from ischemic injury, and in transplanted cadaveric kidneys, it has been demonstrated to reduce delayed graft function.[20]

Furosemide, by blocking the Na^+/K^+ pump in the ascending limb of the Loop of Henle, may prevent oliguric renal failure. No difference in immediate graft function or function at 1 year could be seen between the use of mannitol or furosemide and no diuretic at all.[27]

Use of renal dose dopamine (2–3 µg/kg/min) has been questioned because denervated renal transplants do not respond to dopamine-like native kidneys. No improvement was shown in graft function, and length of intensive care unit (ICU) stay was prolonged in patients receiving dopamine infusions.[28] A small study by Sorbello and colleagues[29] compared dopamine versus fenoldopam infusion (a selective dopamine receptor type 1 [DA-1] agonist) in living donor renal transplantation. Significant improvement in postoperative renal function (diuresis and electrolyte excretion) was seen with fenoldopam. Further rigorous randomized controlled trials are needed to clarify this effect.

Brauer and colleagues[30] investigated whether furosemide, dopamine, and prostaglandin E1 were beneficial in preventing delayed graft function. The investigators demonstrated that renal function was actually worse in the intervention group (with higher urea and creatinine levels).

Emergence

At the conclusion of surgery, muscle relaxation should be reversed and the patient should be extubated if appropriate. Postoperative ICU admission in patients undergoing renal transplant is unusual (<1% in one case series), most commonly occurring because of fluid overload, respiratory distress, or infectious complications.[31] Postoperative pain is typically of mild to moderate intensity and frequently controlled with fentanyl titrated to effect, followed by patient-controlled analgesia (PCA).

The Living Donor

Living donors are intensively screened before surgery.[32] Donor health assessment can significantly prolong the time from organ requirement to donation but is necessary to prevent harm to an otherwise healthy patient. As such donors are almost exclusively healthy ASA 1 or 2 patients.

Surgical technique has moved away from the traditional "open" approach to the laparoscopic hand-assisted donor nephrectomy. The latter technique has the advantage of reducing postoperative pain, allowing earlier mobilization and a shorter hospital stay. Graft function and safety has been shown to be comparable to organs harvested via open nephrectomy.[33]

Induction

Standard ASA monitoring is sufficient for most donor nephrectomies. Anesthesia is induced with IV propofol, judicious opioid use, and neuromuscular blockade. Endotracheal intubation is then performed. The patient is then positioned in the lateral position with a break in the table to allow surgical access. Either kidney may be used; however, the left kidney is preferable because of a longer vascular pedicle. Meticulous care must be taken to prevent pressure areas or nerve injury.

Maintenance

Anesthesia is usually maintained with volatile anesthetic agents, and care is taken to ensure deep neuromuscular blockade to prevent damage to vascular structures while organ harvest is performed.

Fluid management

Care is taken to ensure adequate renal perfusion and urine production during surgery so as to optimize graft function posttransplantation. The pneumoperitoneum established during laparoscopic surgery has adverse effects on hemodynamics, reducing cardiac output and renal perfusion. Often, generous volumes of IV crystalloid are infused to ensure adequate kidney perfusion and to stimulate urine production, typically 10 to 20 mL/kg/h. Mertens zur Borg and colleagues[34] demonstrated that overnight IV hydration before surgery followed by intraoperative colloid bolus administration improved intraoperative urine output and stroke volumes when compared with aggressive intraoperative fluid administration alone.

Direct-acting vasopressor agents should be avoided if possible to prevent graft vasoconstriction. If required, dopamine or low-dose ephedrine should be used for hemodynamic support.

In many institutions, the surgical team, in addition to providing a target for fluid loading, also asks for the administration of diuretics to promote urine production. Typically, furosemide, 20 mg, as a bolus, and mannitol, 12.5 g, are given to improve diuresis. Before clamping of the renal vasculature, 3000 to 5000 units of heparin are administered to prevent coagulation in the graft, which is commonly reversed with protamine after harvest of the kidney.

Laparoscopic donor nephrectomy is typically not unduly painful and does not warrant the use of epidural catheter insertion. Intraoperative pain relief is provided with a balanced simple analgesic and opioid technique. Fentanyl is most commonly used and is titrated to effect. Transversus abdominal plane (TAP) block has been shown to be efficacious in this setting. Parikh and colleagues[35] demonstrated a prolonged analgesic effect and reduced requirement for breakthrough pain relief with ultrasound-guided TAP block.

Postoperative care can be provided in the postanesthetic care unit except in rare circumstances.

LIVER TRANSPLANTATION
Brief Overview

Liver transplantation has become the treatment of choice for eligible patients with end-stage liver disease (ESLD) and has overall excellent outcomes with a nationwide 5-year graft survival rate of over 70%.[36] Most liver transplants are isolated liver transplants from deceased donors. Transplantations of split liver grafts or pared down grafts as well as living donor transplants or transplantation of organs recovered donation after cardiac death (DCD) represent only a small fraction of the volume. Also, combined liver-kidney transplantation is performed only infrequently because patient and graft survival are inferior when compared with single-organ transplantation.[37]

Transplant Recipient—Anesthetic Management

The anesthetic management for liver transplants may be standardized at each liver transplant center, but it varies widely between centers. The management highly depends on the surgical approach (bicaval cross-clamp, piggyback, or venovenous bypass [VVBP]), on the experience of surgeons and anesthesiologists, as well as on the case volume. In a survey of 62 transplant centers in the United States performed by Schumann,[38] a pulmonary artery catheter was used in approximately 30%, transesophageal echocardiography (TEE) in 11.3%, and VVBP in roughly half of adult transplants. A tendency toward decreased use of pulmonary artery catheters and VVBP was shown with increasing case volume. Similarly, the intraoperative resource and personnel utilization also varies widely between liver transplant centers and is influenced by the same factors.

Anesthetic Choice

Because no anesthetic technique has been established as optimal, balanced techniques using volatile anesthetics in an oxygen/air mixture and opioids as well as IV techniques with combination of opioids, benzodiazepines, and propofol have been used successfully for liver transplantation. With the exception of halothane, all volatile anesthetics are suitable for liver transplantation. Isoflurane and desflurane are the most frequently used. Nitrous oxide should not be used to avoid intestinal distention. The use of epidural catheters is discouraged in this type of procedure because a severe and prolonged perioperative coagulopathy may persist.

Monitoring

In addition to the standard ASA monitors, invasive arterial blood pressure should be measured. This monitoring will also allow measurement of levels of arterial blood gases, blood glucose, and electrolytes (sodium, potassium, and ionized calcium) and the hematocrit value, which is considered routine in most transplant centers. Additional hemodynamic monitoring may consist of pulmonary artery catheter, TEE, simple CVP monitoring, or a combination with the choice being determined by institutional practice. Although guidelines have generally improved preoperative assessment of pulmonary hypertension, there may still be cases with inadequate workup or suspicion for newly developed or worsened pulmonary hypertension prompting placement of a pulmonary artery catheter for preincision diagnostics.[39,40]

Recently, TEE has been used more frequently for fluid management, monitoring of cardiac function, and identification of intraoperative complications (eg, pulmonary embolus). Transfusion to correct severe coagulopathy may be considered before line placement, but there are no generally accepted guidelines for this patient population, especially because the use of ultrasound guidance for central vein cannulation has become the standard of care.

Electrolyte, acid-base, and metabolic derangements as well as significant blood loss and coagulopathy are monitored with frequent intraoperative blood samples for point-of-care and laboratory testing. Aside from guiding transfusion and interventions to correct other derangements, monitoring of base deficits and lactate levels after reperfusion of the new graft can be used to assess function of the donor liver. Although considerable controversy exists regarding the benefits of using thrombelastography or similar techniques to monitor coagulation during liver transplantation, like other point-of-care tests, it provides faster results than the average laboratory turnaround time for coagulation studies.

Vascular Access

Line placement should include a radial arterial line for invasive blood pressure monitoring, some form of central venous access, and 2 to 3 large-bore IV catheters, ideally including a rapid-infusion catheter. As mentioned before, the choices for central and large-bore peripheral venous access are highly variable between institutions. Similarly, practices for arterial access differ widely between transplant centers with some placing femoral arterial lines or routinely placing 2 arterial lines.

Induction and Maintenance

Patients selected for liver transplantation usually have preserved cardiac function, although the cardiovascular physiology in ESLD is significantly altered with often severe peripheral vasodilation and increased cardiac output. However, it is usually not necessary to place an arterial line or a central line/pulmonary artery catheter for invasive monitoring before induction. Because ascites, encephalopathy, or uremia frequently present in ESLD, cricoid pressure and RSI should be strongly considered. Induction can be accomplished with any IV anesthetic such as propofol or etomidate, with or without opioids. The choice of opioid depends on institutional preference, and several drugs such as fentanyl, sufentanil, or remifentanil have been used successfully. A short- or intermediate-acting neuromuscular blocking agent should be used to facilitate endotracheal intubation. Given the reduced peripheral vascular resistance in ESLD, hypotension after induction is common and can mostly be treated with administration of small boluses of vasoconstrictors (eg, phenylephrine). An orogastric tube should be placed to improve surgical exposure through decompression of the stomach. The benefit of placing of a nasogastric tube, if desired, should be carefully weighed against the risk of bleeding in the setting of coagulopathy. Before the incision is made, appropriate antibiotic coverage should be ensured.

Pharmacokinetics and pharmacodynamics are significantly altered in ESLD affecting the action of drugs commonly used in anesthesia including benzodiazepines and nondepolarizing neuromuscular blockers. It is very difficult to predict the pharmacokinetics and pharmacodynamics of any given drug in the setting of liver transplantation because the dysfunctional native liver is going to be removed and replaced by a new graft. Initial graft function is difficult to predict and measure, and only secondary indicators such as lactate levels are available to assess function. However, in the case of neuromuscular blockers, it seems reasonable to choose cisatracurium and atracurium because they are cleared independently of liver function.[41]

Fluid Management and Transfusion

The surgical procedure can be divided into 3 major parts, dissection phase, anhepatic phase, and reperfusion phase. It is useful to consider these different phases when thinking about specific goals of fluid administration and hemodynamics. The surgical approach (bicaval clamp, piggyback, or VVBP) also has a major impact on fluid and hemodynamic management.

In general, close communication with the blood bank before and during surgery is crucial. A standard protocol should be established that will guide the setup for blood products. While center volume and experience play a major role, a typical setup may include 10 units of packed red blood cells (PRBC) and 10 units of fresh frozen plasma (FFP) to be brought to the operating room, with 4 units of single-donor platelets available on request. A high-volume transfusion device is typically used and should be connected to a large-bore IV line. These devices include efficient warming systems that will help together with other fluid warmers and warming blankets to maintain the patient's temperature as close to normal as possible.

The fluid requirement during a liver transplantation is significant because of bleeding and fluid shifts. In addition to blood products from the blood bank, the use of intraoperative cell salvage is common unless there are contraindications (eg, malignancy). Furthermore, most centers use a combination of crystalloid (preferred is normal saline) and colloid (preferred is albumin) to maintain intravascular volume. The practices in US transplant centers have recently been surveyed and results published by Schumann and coworkers.[42]

Early in the dissection phase, acute decompression of ascites frequently unmasks intravascular volume depletion and might result in significant hypotension. Adequate volume replacement before or in addition to vasoconstrictor use is crucial at that time. Unless anemia and/or coagulopathy are also present, colloids are frequently the first choice for fluid therapy at that time. Overall, during the dissection, relative normovolemia should be maintained while replacing blood loss and avoiding excessive dilution of coagulation factors. Depending on the underlying cause of the liver disease and the degree of portal hypertension, bleeding can vary dramatically from minimal in some patients to severe blood loss at the other end of the spectrum.

As mentioned earlier, the utilization of VVBP during the anhepatic phase to improve hemodynamic stability as opposed to a bicaval clamp without bypass is center dependent. Some transplant centers use VVBP routinely, whereas others routinely proceed without it. The risk-benefit assessment probably depends on training, expertise, and volume. Based on a study by Schwarz and colleagues,[43] the outcome (mortality, graft function, and kidney function) is not different between a group with a drop in cardiac output of more than 50% after caval clamping and a group with a less-pronounced effect, arguing that VVBP might not provide any outcome advantage even if the cardiac output can be better maintained. Recently, the use of the piggyback technique seems to become more popular with good outcomes. Using this approach, the inferior vena cava is only partially occluded during the anhepatic phase allowing improved venous return and better hemodynamics, although the surgical technique might be more difficult and may lead to more complications.[44,45]

The dissection ends and the anhepatic phase begins with excision of the native liver and control of bleeding. The ice-cold liver donor graft is placed into the surgical field after being flushed to remove the organ preservation solution. The suprahepatic and infrahepatic caval and portal vein anastomoses are then completed in that order. In the piggyback approach, only one caval anastomosis needs to be completed. The hepatic artery anastomosis is often performed after restoration of blood flow.

Before the anhepatic phase, especially when a complete caval occlusion is anticipated, a combination of products as indicated by blood count and coagulation parameters should be infused to increase the patient's intravascular volume and preload so that partial or total caval occlusion and portal vein occlusion are better tolerated. A target CVP between 10 and 20 mm Hg should be achieved to minimize hemodynamic instability when complete occlusion of the vena cava is used. The surgeons should perform a test clamp so that the hemodynamic impact can be better anticipated and the fluid and vasoconstrictor therapy can be optimized before the anhepatic phase. One should avoid aggressive fluid administration during this phase because of possible fluid overload after release of the clamps.

In addition to monitoring laboratory values to assess coagulation, close attention should be paid to the surgical field. Laboratory parameters will be helpful in the underlying mechanism for the coagulopathy (dilution/consumption of clotting factors, platelet entrapment, endogenous heparinoid-like substances, and primary fibrinolysis), but moderate abnormalities in laboratory parameters should probably not be treated in the absence of clinical bleeding with the possibility of a rapid trend to abnormal values. One difficulty in the assessment is the slow turnaround time for laboratory tests. The approach to correct coagulopathy and achieve hemostasis in the absence of surgical bleeding depends on the method of coagulation monitoring and institutional preference. However, the administration of PRBC, FFP, platelets, and cryoprecipitate seems to remain the preferred method to treat blood loss and coagulopathy during liver transplantation.[42]

Postsurgical care of the patient undergoing liver transplant is generally in the ICU, although selected patients (eg, after transplant for hepatocellular carcinoma) may be candidates for an intermediate care setting depending on the setup. Extubation in the operating room is possible in a large percentage of patients depending on volume and experience in the transplant center.

Hemodynamic Management

Patients with ESLD often have very low peripheral vascular resistance and high cardiac output, which may be associated with intravascular volume depletion, especially in the setting of refractory ascites. Patients frequently present with a low normal blood pressure or even with hypotension and may require blood pressure support as early as during induction. Careful attention should be paid to ensure adequate fluid therapy in addition to vasoconstrictor therapy. Commonly used agents are phenylephrine and norepinephrine as well as vasopressin, mostly in combination. Dopamine and dobutamine are also used but less frequently.[42] Phenylephrine is the most common drug administered as bolus.[42] Vasopressor support often increases significantly during the anhepatic phase, especially when complete caval occlusion is used. As mentioned earlier, a temporary "test clamp" on the inferior vena cava may help guide management before vascular clamps are permanently placed for the anhepatic stage. If VVBP is used to blunt the hemodynamic consequences of vascular exclusion, bypass is usually accomplished by cannulation of the femoral and portal veins with diversion to the suprahepatic vena cava through the axillary, subclavian, or jugular vein.[46]

At the end of the anhepatic phase, with the release of the vascular clamps, the preload improves after establishing unobstructed flow in the inferior vena cava and hemodynamics usually improves. The removal of the portal vein clamp marks the beginning of reperfusion. Blood from the splanchnic circulation perfuses the new donor liver. This part of the operation is often the most critical from an anesthesia management perspective because significant hemodynamic instability and cardiac arrest may occur immediately after reperfusion.[47] Manifestation can include various problems such as decreased inotropy leading to profound hypotension, severely decreased chronotropy leading to arrhythmias or full arrest, as well as hyperkalemic arrest. Anesthetic management is directed at maintaining or recovering cardiovascular stability.[48] This goal may require immediate pharmacologic intervention such as the administration of epinephrine, atropine, calcium, or occasionally sodium bicarbonate. In severe cases, methylene blue might be considered because it has been shown to attenuate hemodynamic changes of the reperfusion syndrome.[49] Preoperative placement of external pacing/defibrillation pads may be helpful in cases of immediate postreperfusion cardiac arrest.

Discussion of Adjuvant Drugs

Octreotide as infusion can be used intraoperatively for the treatment of severe portal hypertension with the goal to reduce portal pressure and bleeding.

Ionized calcium levels can be significantly decreased during liver transplantation, especially when large volumes of PRBC and/or FFP need to be transfused. The citrate load from these products can lead to significantly reduced calcium levels, in particular during the anhepatic phase when even the remaining capacity to metabolize citrate is removed.[50] Administration of calcium chloride or calcium gluconate as infusion or bolus is often required, and calcium levels should be regularly monitored.

In addition, the glucose-insulin pathway is frequently impaired in patients with ESLD, and close monitoring of blood glucose levels is required. Administration of steroids for immunosuppression, enhanced glycogenolysis, and insulin resistance of the graft may all contribute to hyperglycemia requiring insulin treatment.[50] Close monitoring of electrolytes is also essential, and hypo- or hyperkalemia are not uncommon and often require treatment. Interventions used for renal protection have not been shown to provide improved outcomes.[51] One possible benefit of diuretics despite lack of renal protection may be the promotion of diuresis, which could make volume management easier especially if coagulopathy needs to be treated.

Immunosuppressive therapy is crucial for the success of transplantation. Protocols vary between medical centers, and clear communication is crucial for intraoperative delivery of the appropriate immunosuppressant (eg, steroid).

Several drugs, such as aprotinin, tranexamic acid, aminocaproic acid, and recombinant factor VIIa (rFVIIa) have been used in liver transplantation to reduce transfusion requirements. The efficacy of these approaches from the view of a starting liver transplant program with an emphasis on affordability has recently been reviewed by Rando and coworkers.[52] Caution seems to be advised, especially in patients at risk for thrombotic complications because a dose that effectively reduces blood loss may at the same time increase the risk for hepatic artery or portal vein thrombosis or other thrombotic complications. However, most evidence exists for a benefit of the use of tranexamic acid. In addition, rFVIIa, initially developed for the treatment of patients with hemophilia, has been advocated for use in liver transplantation among other surgical settings. Given the high cost of rFVIIa and the lack of benefit demonstrated in prospective randomized trials, routine use in liver transplantation cannot be recommended.[52–54] However, there is probably enough data from case reports and series as well as noncontrolled trials that it is reasonable to consider rFVIIa in extreme situations.[52,55]

The Living Donor

The first successful liver transplants from living donors were reported almost 25 years ago and are today performed as adult-to-child and adult-to-adult transplants.[56] The regenerative capacity of the liver allows for complete recovery in donor and recipient after both a left or right lobe transplant. The choice between right or left hepatectomy is made depending on the relation between size of the recipient and the estimated mass of the donor lobe.

Induction

Living donors are thoroughly screened preoperatively and are ASA 1 or 2 patients without any medical problem, which would significantly increase their anesthetic or surgical risk. Otherwise, the considerations for anesthetic management of the donor are similar to those of patients undergoing hepatectomies. Preoperative placement of a thoracic epidural catheter for postoperative pain control is performed in some transplant centers, whereas others rely on PCA. A recent study argues that pain control is better with an epidural technique compared with PCA and that concerns about safety based on possible coagulopathy may not seem to be justified.[57,58]

A standard IV induction can be performed using any IV anesthetic and neuromuscular blocker of choice. Intraoperatively, the patient is placed in a supine position, frequently with one arm tucked (right or left) at the side and the other abducted. Two large-bore IV catheters and invasive arterial blood pressure monitoring are used in most centers.[59,60] An orogastric tube should be placed to improve surgical exposure through decompression of the stomach.

Maintenance

The intraoperative care of patients undergoing donor hepatectomy for liver donation is similar to that of other patients having other hepatic surgery. General anesthesia is standard and may consist of a balanced technique or be combined with intraoperative supplementation of epidural analgesia. Paralysis is maintained throughout the operation. While the liver is mobilized, there may be brief periods of hypotension because of temporary decrease in venous return to the heart. These episodes usually do not require treatment especially because the donors are usually healthy.

Fluid management

Intravenous fluid is administered cautiously until the graft has been isolated. This technique is generally advocated to maintain a low CVP to help minimize blood loss during transection.[61] However, in a retrospective study, CVP monitoring did not seem to reduce blood loss when compared with patients without CVP monitoring. Fluid restriction without measuring the CVP seems to be sufficient.[62] Although blood loss at most centers is usually well below 1000 mL, the nature of the procedure warrants vigilance and preparation.[63] Therefore, liver donors usually donate 1 or 2 autologous units of blood before surgery. In addition, intraoperative cell salvage is utilized at most centers.

In most cases, the patient can be extubated in the operating room and transferred to the postoperative care unit, and ICU admission is rarely necessary. Nevertheless, in some institutions, living liver donors are routinely managed in the ICU during the early postoperative period.

PANCREAS TRANSPLANTATION

Successful pancreas transplantation can cure patients with diabetic mellitus. Pancreas transplant is frequently performed with simultaneous kidney transplantation, as nephropathy is extremely common in these patients. Recent advances in immunosuppressive therapy have allowed long-term graft survival to be possible. Long-term graft survival had been a significant problem because pancreatic grafts are a potent immunologic trigger.[64]

Intraoperative Management

Pancreas transplant is usually performed under general anesthesia with endotracheal intubation. Surgical duration and the need for stable hemodynamics make a balanced general anesthetic the best choice. Full muscle relaxation is necessary to optimize surgical access. Patients with concurrent renal failure should be paralyzed in a similar way to those undergoing isolated kidney transplant, that is, the use of muscle relaxants that do not rely on renal excretion for the offset of action for maintenance of neuromuscular blockade. Cisatracurium infusion with train-of-four monitoring is the usual practice for these long cases, although intermittent vecuronium boluses have been successfully used.[65] Patients undergoing isolated pancreas transplant (who have reasonable renal function) may be administered any nondepolarizing muscle relaxant provided the depth of blockade is monitored.

In addition to standard ASA monitoring, arterial and central venous line insertion are necessary. RSI is often indicated in this patient cohort. Diabetic gastropathy, secondary to autonomic dysfunction, puts these patients at a high risk of aspiration at induction of anesthesia. Nonparticulate antacid and cricoid pressure should be used.

An epidural catheter can be inserted before induction for intraoperative and postoperative analgesia. Postoperative pain can be significant because of the extensive abdominal exposure required for surgery.

Immunosuppressant and antimicrobial medication is administered in the operating room by the anesthesiologist after induction; clear communication with the surgical team is necessary.

During surgery, careful attention must be paid to maintaining adequate perfusion pressure to optimize graft function. Invasive monitoring allows for close control of hemodynamics and cardiac filling pressures and also permits the ability to draw laboratory tests and arterial blood gas (ABGs). Monitoring the blood glucose level is of paramount importance. Before unclamping of the transplanted pancreas, blood glucose levels must be measure every hour along with monitoring for ketoacidosis. Insulin infusion should be instituted if blood sugar levels become deranged. Hyperglycemia is associated with worsened immune function and increases the risk of infection. After unclamping of the pancreas, glucose levels should be measured every 30 minutes because the blood glucose level typically falls by 50 mg/dL/h.

Autonomic neuropathy may increase the risk of cardiovascular instability under anesthesia; however, a study in uremic renal transplant recipients with diabetes and known autonomic dysfunction failed to illustrate any difference in hemodynamics when compared with uremic nondiabetic patients.[66]

Protracted surgery with extensive abdominal exposure results in significant insensible fluid losses. Choice and volume of fluid administration can be challenging and should be guided by central venous pressures, arterial pulse pressure variation, or where indicated, TEE. Blood products should be administered where necessary to optimize oxygen carriage or to correct coagulopathy. Crystalloid administration should probably be minimized; pancreatic edema seems to be less when colloids are given, although no trial data exists.

INTESTINAL TRANSPLANTATION

Intestinal transplantation is rarely performed, and its predominant indication is short gut syndrome, which accounts for 60% of cases.[67] This technique can be performed as an isolated procedure or combined with simultaneous liver transplantation.

Graft failure is common, although long-term function has improved dramatically with newer immunosuppression. The 1-year graft survival is now 66%, whereas only one-fifth of grafts continue to function at 5 years.

No published trials exist regarding intraoperative anesthetic management and outcome.

REFERENCES

1. Ricaurte L, Vargas J, Lozano E, et al. Anesthesia and kidney transplantation. Transplant Proc 2013;45(4):1386–91.
2. Gaston RS, Alveranga DY, Becker BN, et al. Kidney and pancreas transplantation. Am J Transplant 2003;3(Suppl 4):64–77.
3. Hrabac B, Stranjak M, Hodzić S. The effect of suxamethonium chloride on serum potassium levels during kidney transplantation. Arh Hig Rada Toksikol 1991;42(3):303–7.
4. Turitto VT, Weiss HJ. Red blood cells: their dual role in thrombus formation. Science 1980;207(4430):541–3.
5. Group PS, Devereaux PJ, Yang H, et al. Effects of extended-release metoprolol succinate in patients undergoing non-cardiac surgery (POISE trial): a randomised controlled trial. Lancet 2008;371(9627):1839–47.
6. London MJ, Hur K, Schwartz GG, et al. Association of perioperative β-blockade with mortality and cardiovascular morbidity following major noncardiac surgery. JAMA 2013;309(16):1704–13.
7. Auron M, Harte B, Kumar A, et al. Renin-angiotensin system antagonists in the perioperative setting: clinical consequences and recommendations for practice. Postgrad Med J 2011;87(1029):472–81.

8. Bhosale G, Shah V. Combined spinal-epidural anesthesia for renal transplantation. Transplant Proc 2008;40(4):1122–4.

9. Vandam LD, Harrison JH, Murray JE, et al. Anesthetic aspects of renal homotransplantation in man. With notes on the anesthetic care of the uremic patient. Anesthesiology 1962;23:783–92.

10. Linke CL, Merin RG. A regional anesthetic approach for renal transplantation. Anesth Analg 1976;55(1):69–73.

11. Akpek E, Kayhan Z, Kaya H, et al. Epidural anesthesia for renal transplantation: a preliminary report. Transplant Proc 1999;31(8):3149–50.

12. Modesti C, Sacco T, Morelli G, et al. Balanced anesthesia versus total intravenous anesthesia for kidney transplantation. Minerva Anestesiol 2006;72(7–8):627–35.

13. Kirvelä M, Olkkola KT, Rosenberg PH, et al. Pharmacokinetics of propofol and haemodynamic changes during induction of anaesthesia in uraemic patients. Br J Anaesth 1992;68(2):178–82.

14. Park JH, Lee JH, Joo DJ, et al. Effect of sevoflurane on grafted kidney function in renal transplantation. Korean J Anesthesiol 2012;62(6):529–35.

15. Conzen PF, Kharasch ED, Czerner SFA, et al. Low-flow sevoflurane compared with low-flow isoflurane anesthesia in patients with stable renal insufficiency. Anesthesiology 2002;97(3):578–84.

16. Campos L, Parada B, Furriel F, et al. Do intraoperative hemodynamic factors of the recipient influence renal graft function? Transplant Proc 2012;44(6):1800–3.

17. Hadimioglu N, Ertug Z, Yegin A, et al. Correlation of peripheral venous pressure and central venous pressure in kidney recipients. Transplant Proc 2006;38(2):440–2.

18. Heino A, Orko R, Rosenberg PH. Anaesthesiological complications in renal transplantation: a retrospective study of 500 transplantations. Acta Anaesthesiol Scand 1986;30(7):574–80.

19. Della Rocca G, Pompei L, Coccia C, et al. Atracurium, cisatracurium, vecuronium and rocuronium in patients with renal failure. Minerva Anestesiol 2003;69(7–8):605–11, 612, 5.

20. Koning OH, Ploeg RJ, Van Bockel JH, et al. Risk factors for delayed graft function in cadaveric kidney transplantation: a prospective study of renal function and graft survival after preservation with University of Wisconsin solution in multi-organ donors. European Multicenter Study Group. Transplantation 1997;63(11):1620–8.

21. Ryan DW. Preoperative serum cholinesterase concentration in chronic renal failure. Clinical experience of suxamethonium in 81 patients undergoing renal transplant. Br J Anaesth 1977;49(9):945–9.

22. Goyal P, Puri GD, Pandey CK, et al. Evaluation of induction doses of propofol: comparison between endstage renal disease and normal renal function patients. Anaesth Intensive Care 2002;30(5):584–7.

23. Dawidson I, Berglin E, Brynger H, et al. Intravascular volumes and colloid dynamics in relation to fluid management in living related kidney donors and recipients. Crit Care Med 1987;15(7):631–6.

24. O'Malley CM, Frumento RJ, Bennett-Guerrero E. Intravenous fluid therapy in renal transplant recipients: results of a US survey. Transplant Proc 2002;34(8):3142–5.

25. O'Malley CM, Frumento RJ, Hardy MA, et al. A randomized, double-blind comparison of lactated Ringer's solution and 0.9% NaCl during renal transplantation. Anesth Analg 2005;100(5):1518–24 table of contents.

26. Gabriëls G, August C, Grisk O, et al. Impact of renal transplantation on small vessel reactivity. Transplantation 2003;75(5):689–97.
27. Hanif F, Macrae AN, Littlejohn MG, et al. Outcome of renal transplantation with and without intra-operative diuretics. Int J Surg 2011;9(6):460–3.
28. Ciapetti M, Di Valvasone S, Di Filippo A, et al. Low-dose dopamine in kidney transplantation. Transplant Proc 2009;41(10):4165–8.
29. Sorbello M, Morello G, Paratore A, et al. Fenoldopam vs dopamine as a nephroprotective strategy during living donor kidney transplantation: preliminary data. Transplant Proc 2007;39(6):1794–6.
30. Brauer RB, Marx T, Ulm K, et al. Effect of perioperative administration of a drug regimen on the primary function of human renal allografts. Transplant Proc 2010; 42(5):1523–5.
31. Kogan A, Singer P, Cohen J, et al. Readmission to an intensive care unit following liver and kidney transplantation: a 50-month study. Transplant Proc 1999;31(4):1892–3.
32. Perlis N, Connelly M, D'A Honey JR, et al. Evaluating potential live-renal donors: causes for rejection, deferral and planned procedure type, a single-centre experience. Can Urol Assoc J 2013;7(1–2):41–5.
33. Kok NF, Lind MY, Hansson BM, et al. Comparison of laparoscopic and mini incision open donor nephrectomy: single blind, randomised controlled clinical trial. BMJ 2006;333(7561):221.
34. Mertens zur Borg IR, Kok NF, Lambrou G, et al. Beneficial effects of a new fluid regime on kidney function of donor and recipient during laparoscopic v open donor nephrectomy. J Endourol 2007;21(12):1509–15.
35. Parikh BK, Waghmare VT, Shah VR, et al. The analgesic efficacy of ultrasound-guided transversus abdominis plane block for retroperitoneoscopic donor nephrectomy: a randomized controlled study. Saudi J Anaesth 2013;7(1):43–7.
36. Kim WR, Stock PG, Smith JM, et al. OPTN/SRTR 2011 Annual Data Report: liver. Am J Transplant 2013;13(Suppl 1):73–102.
37. Davis CL, Gonwa TA, Wilkinson AH. Identification of patients best suited for combined liver-kidney transplantation: part II. Liver Transpl 2002;8(3): 193–211.
38. Schumann R. Intraoperative resource utilization in anesthesia for liver transplantation in the United States: a survey. Anesth Analg 2003;97(1):21–8 table of contents.
39. Krowka MJ, Mandell MS, Ramsay MA, et al. Hepatopulmonary syndrome and portopulmonary hypertension: a report of the multicenter liver transplant database. Liver Transpl 2004;10(2):174–82.
40. Krowka MJ, Wiesner RH, Heimbach JK. Pulmonary contraindications, indications and MELD exceptions for liver transplantation: a contemporary view and look forward. J Hepatol 2013;59(2):367–74.
41. De Wolf AM, Freeman JA, Scott VL, et al. Pharmacokinetics and pharmacodynamics of cisatracurium in patients with end-stage liver disease undergoing liver transplantation. Br J Anaesth 1996;76(5):624–8.
42. Schumann R, Mandell S, Michaels MD, et al. Intraoperative fluid and pharmacologic management and the anesthesiologist's supervisory role for nontraditional technologies during liver transplantation: a survey of US Academic Centers. Transplant Proc 2013;45(6):2258–62.
43. Schwarz B, Pomaroli A, Hoermann C, et al. Liver transplantation without venovenous bypass: morbidity and mortality in patients with greater than 50% reduction in cardiac output after vena cava clamping. J Cardiothorac Vasc Anesth 2001;15(4):460–2.

44. Donataccio M, Ruzzenente A, Pachera S, et al. Caval anastomosis in liver transplantation: prospective experience of Verona liver transplantation program. Transplant Proc 2005;37(6):2605–6.

45. Parrilla P, Sanchez-Bueno F, Figueras J, et al. Analysis of the complications of the piggy-back technique in 1112 liver transplants. Transplant Proc 1999; 31(6):2388–9.

46. Tisone G, Mercadante E, Dauri M, et al. Surgical versus percutaneous technique for veno-venous bypass during orthotopic liver transplantation: a prospective randomized study. Transplant Proc 1999;31(8):3162–3.

47. Aggarwal S, Kang Y, Freeman JA, et al. Postreperfusion syndrome: cardiovascular collapse following hepatic reperfusion during liver transplantation. Transplant Proc 1987;19(4 Suppl 3):54–5.

48. Webster NR, Bellamy MC, Lodge JP, et al. Haemodynamics of liver reperfusion: comparison of two anaesthetic techniques. Br J Anaesth 1994;72(4):418–21.

49. Koelzow H, Gedney JA, Baumann J, et al. The effect of methylene blue on the hemodynamic changes during ischemia reperfusion injury in orthotopic liver transplantation. Anesth Analg 2002;94(4):824–9 table of contents.

50. Merritt WT. Metabolism and liver transplantation: review of perioperative issues. Liver Transpl 2000;(4 Suppl 1):S76–84.

51. Zacharias M, Gilmore IC, Herbison GP, et al. Interventions for protecting renal function in the perioperative period. Cochrane Database Syst Rev 2005;(3):CD003590.

52. Rando K, Niemann CU, Taura P, et al. Optimizing cost-effectiveness in perioperative care for liver transplantation: a model for low- to medium-income countries. Liver Transpl 2011;17(11):1247–78.

53. Lodge JP, Jonas S, Jones RM, et al. Efficacy and safety of repeated perioperative doses of recombinant factor VIIa in liver transplantation. Liver Transpl 2005; 11(8):973–9.

54. Planinsic RM, Van der Meer J, Testa G, et al. Safety and efficacy of a single bolus administration of recombinant factor VIIa in liver transplantation due to chronic liver disease. Liver Transpl 2005;11(8):895–900.

55. Niemann CU, Behrends M, Quan D, et al. Recombinant factor VIIa reduces transfusion requirements in liver transplant patients with high MELD scores. Transfus Med 2006;16(2):93–100.

56. Samstein B, Emond J. Liver transplants from living related donors. Annu Rev Med 2001;52:147–60.

57. Choi SJ, Gwak MS, Ko JS, et al. The changes in coagulation profile and epidural catheter safety for living liver donors: a report on 6 years of our experience. Liver Transpl 2007;13(1):62–70.

58. Clarke H, Chandy T, Srinivas C, et al. Epidural analgesia provides better pain management after live liver donation: a retrospective study. Liver Transpl 2011;17(3):315–23.

59. Adachi T. Anesthetic principles in living-donor liver transplantation at Kyoto University Hospital: experiences of 760 cases. J Anesth 2003;17(2):116–24.

60. Niemann CU, Roberts JP, Ascher NL, et al. Intraoperative hemodynamics and liver function in adult-to-adult living liver donors. Liver Transpl 2002;8(12):1126–32.

61. Melendez JA, Arslan V, Fischer ME, et al. Perioperative outcomes of major hepatic resections under low central venous pressure anesthesia: blood loss, blood transfusion, and the risk of postoperative renal dysfunction. J Am Coll Surg 1998;187(6):620–5.

62. Niemann CU, Feiner J, Behrends M, et al. Central venous pressure monitoring during living right donor hepatectomy. Liver Transpl 2007;13(2):266–71.

63. Lutz JT, Valentin-Gamazo C, Gorlinger K, et al. Blood-transfusion requirements and blood salvage in donors undergoing right hepatectomy for living related liver transplantation. Anesth Analg 2003;96(2):351–5 table of contents.
64. Gruessner RW, Bartlett ST, Burke GW, et al. Suggested guidelines for the use of tacrolimus in pancreas/kidney transplantation. Clin Transplant 1998;12(3):260–2.
65. Sakamoto H, Takita K, Kemmotsu O, et al. Increased sensitivity to vecuronium and prolonged duration of its action in patients with end-stage renal failure. J Clin Anesth 2001;13(3):193–7.
66. Kirvela M, Scheinin M, Lindgren L. Haemodynamic and catecholamine responses to induction of anaesthesia and tracheal intubation in diabetic and non-diabetic uraemic patients. Br J Anaesth 1995;74(1):60–5.
67. Roberts JP, Brown RS Jr, Edwards EB, et al. Liver and intestine transplantation. Am J Transplant 2003;3(Suppl 4):78–90.

Postoperative Care/Critical Care of the Transplant Patient

Geraldine C. Diaz, DO[a],*, Gebhard Wagener, MD[b],
John F. Renz, MD, PhD[c]

KEYWORDS

- Solid-organ abdominal transplantation • Complications of abdominal transplantation
- Posttransplant critical care • Early allograft function

KEY POINTS

- Recipient selection criteria for abdominal solid-organ transplantation are being relaxed to increase patient access.
- Donor selection criteria are being relaxed to expand allograft supply.
- Assessment and optimization of early allograft function are the principal goals of critical care.
- Astute surveillance, early diagnosis, and appropriate treatment of postoperative complications improve outcomes.

INTRODUCTION

The notable achievements in organ transplantation since the introduction of effective immunosuppression have dramatically changed the prognosis for patients with renal, hepatic, pancreatic, and intestinal failure.[1–4] General improvements in outcomes of abdominal solid-organ transplant recipients (ASORs) have resulted in relaxation of candidate eligibility criteria and a large increase in the number of patients awaiting an allograft.[5] Since 2000, the percentage of liver and kidney recipients older than 65 years has increased by 84% and 101%, respectively (**Fig. 1**).[5]

Increasing recipient demand has stimulated relaxation of donor selection criteria, creating a unique allograft qualifier termed expanded or marginal.[6,7] Expanded criteria donor (ECD) allografts imply a greater risk of donor transmitted disease or allograft failure.[8,9] These inferior-quality allografts may be suitable for selected recipients

[a] Department of Anesthesia and Critical Care, University of Chicago, 5841 South Maryland Avenue, Chicago, IL 60637, USA; [b] Department of Anesthesiology, Columbia University College of Physicians and Surgeons, 630 West 168th Street, New York, NY 10032, USA; [c] Section of Abdominal Organ Transplantation, Department of Surgery, University of Chicago, 5841 South Maryland Avenue, Chicago, IL 60637, USA
* Corresponding author.
E-mail address: gdiaz@dacc.uchicago.edu

Anesthesiology Clin 31 (2013) 723–735
http://dx.doi.org/10.1016/j.anclin.2013.09.001
1932-2275/13/$ – see front matter © 2013 Elsevier Inc. All rights reserved.

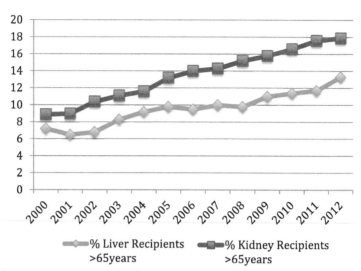

**% Liver Recipients
>65years**   **% Kidney Recipients
>65years**

Fig. 1. The increasing percentage of liver and kidney recipients aged more than 65 years. (*Data from* Scientific Registry of Transplant Recipients, United Network for Organ Sharing.)

who would otherwise wait too long for a standard criteria allograft.[10–12] ECD allografts show a higher incidence of delayed graft function and ischemia/reperfusion injury (IRI) in the immediate postoperative period. As the donor and recipient envelopes expand, the risk to ECD recipients has never been higher, whereas potential consequences from complications in this physiologically fragile recipient group have never been greater.

This article describes the 3 principles germane to the management of ASORs: early assessment of allograft function; optimizing support for the transplanted allograft within the context of the recipient's preexisting conditions; and surveillance, recognition, and management of early postoperative complications.

EARLY ASSESSMENT OF ALLOGRAFT FUNCTION

Understanding the donor, recipient, and intraoperative events is paramount to assessment of early allograft function (EAF). All available donor information, including hemodynamic stability, allograft function at recovery, acidosis, vasopressor utilization, sepsis, biopsy data, concomitant organ-system failure, and any history of organ dysfunction, is essential. The mechanism of recovery (donation after brain death [DBD] or donation after cardiac death [DCD]) has the single largest effect on predicting the function of kidney, liver, pancreas, and intestinal allografts. DBD is the most common recovery technique; however, DCD has recently shown significant growth with the potential to expand the donor pool greatly.[13]

The physiologic changes occurring in DBD and DCD are fundamentally different and poorly understood (**Table 1**).[14] Progression to brain death in DBD is secondary to cerebral insult and mass effect. These intracranial events may or may not be associated with systemic ischemia. Recovery occurs in the presence of continuous organ perfusion within the heart-beating brain-dead donor until it is deliberately interrupted by the surgeon, who instantaneously initiates cold allograft perfusion. Because the donor has been legally declared brain dead, the prerecovery period provides an opportunity for donor resuscitation, optimization of organ function, and clinical assessment through additional laboratories or biopsy, before allocation.[15]

Table 1
Significant clinical differences between DBD and DCD

	DBD	DCD
Death criteria	Neurologic	Cardiopulmonary
Donor conditioning	Yes	Minimal
Intraoperative conditioning	Yes	No
Organ assessment	Before perfusion	After perfusion
Preservation	Immediate	Delayed
Injury pattern	Insult-stabilization-conditioning-recovery	Insult-stabilization-withdraw-ischemia-recovery

Abbreviations: DBD, donation after brain death; DCD, donation after cardiac death.

DCD donors do not fulfill brain death criteria so recovery can only begin after declaration of cardiopulmonary death followed by a variable observation period to exclude spontaneous autoresuscitation.[15] The patient's neurologic status limits resuscitation efforts, precludes invasive procedures to assess organ quality, prevents extensive assessment of end-organ function, and impedes allograft optimization before recovery. Additional ischemic injury follows withdrawal of support and cardiopulmonary arrest at recovery. Organ assessment can only occur after procurement has proceeded through cold perfusion with no opportunity for intraoperative organ resuscitation.[14]

The recipient's intraoperative record should be reviewed for events that accentuate IRI, such as hypotension, vasopressor utilization, acidosis, a failed anastomosis that required revision, thrombosis of an anastomosis, or other technical difficulties that may have prolonged warm ischemia. Substantial differences in the hemodynamic environment between donor and recipient can affect outcome in renal transplantation because allografts from hypertensive donors perform poorly in the setting of recipient hypotension.

In renal transplantation, delayed graft function (DGF) is defined as a requirement for dialysis within 1 week after transplantation.[16] Subsequent studies identified DGF as acute renal failure resulting in posttransplant oliguria, enhanced allograft immunogenicity, an increased risk of acute rejection, and decreased long-term survival.[1,17,18] ECD allografts, by definition, show a greater than or equal to 70% risk of failure compared with standard criteria allografts.[6] ECD donors are defined as greater than or equal to 60 years of age or aged 50 to 59 years with 2 of the following 3 characteristics: cerebrovascular accident as the cause of death, a history of hypertension, or a terminal creatinine of greater than 1.5 mg/dL.[6]

The effect of DGF on long-term renal function depends on recovery technique. DGF is observed more frequently among DCD renal allografts[18,19]; however, DGF does not significantly affect long-term renal function, particularly when the DCD donor was less than 50 years of age and cold ischemia time is limited to less than 12 hours.[19] In DBD, DGF is a significant risk factor for acute rejection, primary nonfunction, chronic renal insufficiency, and decreased graft survival.[1,16,20] DGF in the setting of a DBD or living donor renal allograft warrants an immediate investigation for an underlying vascular cause or complication of rejection.

DGF for extrarenal abdominal allografts is less defined. With regard to liver transplantation, estimation of hepatic allograft function is difficult because it depends on the preoperative patient condition as well. Liver allocation is based on the Model for End-Stage Liver Disease (MELD) score,[21] a disease severity score based on total bilirubin, serum creatinine, and International Normalized Ratio; however, up to 25% of patients receive exceptions whereby their allocation priority MELD is adjusted for specific conditions, such as hepatocellular carcinoma.[22] As a result, liver transplant recipients may range from a noncirrhotic patient diagnosed with alpha-1-antitrypsin deficiency driving in to the hospital from home to a cirrhotic patient intubated in the intensive care unit on vasopressors and hemodialysis. This variability complicates the definition of DGF; however, a recent definition based on bilirubin, transaminases, and International Normalized Ratio has been retrospectively validated, (**Box 1**).[23] Although metabolic demand from the liver cannot be measured directly, metabolic demand can be expected to increase with recipient physiologic MELD, hypothermia, acidosis, large intraoperative blood loss, or past medical history significant for extensive abdominal surgery or retransplantation. If allograft supply cannot satisfy demand or requires extrahepatic support, the allograft is experiencing DGF. If allograft supply plus maximal extrahepatic support cannot satisfy demand, the allograft is showing primary nonfunction. Predictors of DGF include donor age greater than 70 years, cold ischemic time greater than 12 hours, greater than 30% macrovesicular steatosis, DCD, and deteriorating donor physiology at recovery.[7] Donor liver function tests have never been shown to correlate with posttransplant allograft function. MELD score on posttransplant day 5 has recently been shown to be a sensitive predictor of 90-day mortality and allograft failure.[24]

A liver donor risk index (DRI) has been created that incorporates age, cause of death, height, DCD, partial allograft transplantation, and allocation unit as variables in creating a metric to estimate the risk of allograft failure compared with an ideal donor.[25] Although an important first step in creating a metric to quantify allograft risk, the liver DRI is insufficiently powered to be the sole metric in determining allograft suitability.

The surgeon and anesthesiologist should be queried about intraoperative bile production, correction of acidosis, vasopressor requirements, and urine output because these are critical in assessing EAF. Additional early benchmarks include demonstrable mental status, lactic acid clearance, thermoregulation, glucose production, correction of coagulopathy, and preservation of renal function.[26]

EAF in pancreas and small bowel allografts is even less defined. In pancreas and small bowel transplantation, immediate allograft performance is not a physiologic mandate because the principal allograft functions can be temporarily supported.[12,27,28] The risk of these allografts is thrombosis with resulting ischemia and necrosis. The challenge with EAF is to verify function as a marker of allograft viability. Thus, the absence of verified allograft function should prompt an immediate investigation for allograft thrombosis.

Pancreatic and intestinal allografts are low-blood-flow organs with parenchyma that are exquisitely sensitive to ischemia. Pancreatic allografts manifest ischemia as pancreatitis when IRI causes local inflammation that reduces microvascular flow

---

Box 1
Definition of early allograft dysfunction in liver transplant recipients

INR greater than or equal to 1.6 on postoperative day 7

Bilirubin greater than or equal to 10 mg/dL on postoperative day 7

ALT or AST greater than 2000 IU/mL within the first 7 postoperative days

Abbreviations: ALT, alanine aminotransferase; AST, aspartate aminotransferase; INR, International Normalized Ratio.

Adapted from Olthoff K, Kulik L, Samstein B, et al. Validation of a current definition of early allograft dysfunction in liver transplant recipients and analysis of risk factors. Liver Transpl 2010;16:943–9; with permission.

and promotes thrombosis. Thrombosis accelerates parenchymal ischemia leading to necrosis, superinfection, and additional inflammation.[28,29]

Intestinal allografts show ischemic injury through epithelial sloughing with disarray of Langerhans crypts, which stimulates its own immunologic response in addition to pathogen translocation leading to further inflammation and necrosis. The immunologic destruction of the mucosal lining stimulates fibroblast invasion and fibrosis, which further impede intestinal absorption.[12]

Meticulous surgical technique during recovery and allograft preparation is essential to intestinal and pancreatic allograft outcomes. The extensive microvascular beds within intestines and pancreas are sensitive to increased pressure during recovery or excessive volumes of preservation fluid. Donor risk factors associated with allograft thrombosis include increased donor age, hemodynamic instability, catecholamine requirements, and acidosis. Cold ischemia exceeding 12 hours is an additional independent risk factor for technical failure.[28–30]

The appearance and texture of the pancreas on completion of the procedure is essential because pancreatitis and allograft edema are common at reperfusion. In this setting, osmotic diuretics are frequently administered to decrease edema and improve microvascular perfusion. A similar strategy is used with intestinal allografts to limit edema and bowel distention. The failure of an allograft to respond to intraoperative interventions aimed at reducing edema is a signal to maintain astute surveillance of allograft function perioperatively.

OPTIMAL SUPPORT OF THE TRANSPLANTED ALLOGRAFT

Optimizing the recipient's physiology after transplantation yields the greatest chance of organ recovery. In patients with DGF following renal transplantation, immunosuppressive protocols should be continued with standard target drug trough levels.[31] The traditional practice to lower immunosuppression in the setting of DGF for renal transplant patients is not supported by current literature.

Estimation of hepatic EAF is challenging. An essential strategy is that an ounce of prevention is worth a pound of cure because supplementing early hepatic function and deescalating therapies as the allograft shows sufficient function averts large resuscitations for recipient instability. This strategy includes broad-spectrum antibiotics and antifungals targeted against translocation, intubation until mental status is certain, blood product supplementation to avert coagulopathy, and prevention of hypothermia. Early trophic feeding maintains enterocyte health and decreases bacterial translocation while stimulating enterohepatic circulation to improve biliary physiology.[10]

Optimal support for the pancreatic allograft focuses on detection and prevention of thrombosis. Although never scientifically validated, prophylactic anticoagulation involving low-dose systemic heparin in the operating theater with dose escalation through the first week after transplantation supplemented with aspirin therapy is routine.[28] Volume status, particularly in the setting of combined kidney-pancreas transplantation, is critical to avert venous thrombosis because the newly transplanted kidney produces large amounts of urine, particularly when diuretics have been administered to reduce pancreatic edema.[28,29]

Pancreatitis and pancreatic ischemia typically present as abdominal pain, peritonitis, ileus, and fever.[28,32] Serum amylase and lipase correlate poorly with the severity of allograft pancreatitis, whereas prolonged posttransplant hyperamylasemia is observed in more than 30% of recipients[33]; however, trend analysis is helpful. In particular, a sudden increase in amylase and lipase with a change in exogenous insulin requirements is a predictor of graft necrosis. The use of Doppler ultrasound is increasing in popularity. This modality is operator and patient habitus dependent; however, when satisfactory imaging is achieved, Doppler ultrasound is sensitive in diagnosing thrombosis.[34] Computed tomography with contrast angiography has been advocated in the diagnosis of vascular complications; however, the authors prefer surgical exploration to computed tomography because most of these patients also have a transplanted renal allograft.

There are even fewer serum markers and radiologic modalities to guide the management of intestinal transplant recipients. In this population, clinicians only have physical examination, ostomy output, and laboratory analysis for hyperkalemia or metabolic acidosis. As in pancreas recipients, prophylactic anticoagulation is routine; however, appropriate volume resuscitation is even more difficult because volume depletion occurs secondary to inflammation and poor fluid absorption from the transplanted intestine in addition to ileostomy losses.[12,35] The differential diagnosis between metabolic acidosis secondary to IRI and luminal losses of bicarbonate is important because luminal bicarbonate losses can be treated with replacement therapy.[35] Intestinal transplant recipients typically show malnutrition and protein deficiency that results in low oncotic pressure and further loss of intravascular fluids.[35] As in liver transplantation, large bolus-type volume resuscitation should be avoided, whereas goal-directed fluid and electrolyte therapy achieves a balanced physiology. Preserving the integrity of the intestinal villi requires early nutritional support through trophic feeding of dilute glucose-containing formulas. As intestinal motility is restored, enteral feedings can be accelerated.

RECOGNITION AND MANAGEMENT OF EARLY COMPLICATIONS
Infectious Complications

Posttransplant infections include bacteremia, fungemia, pneumonia, wound infection, intra-abdominal fluid collections, urinary infections, and *Clostridium difficile* colitis.[36] Prophylactic antimicrobial and antiviral therapies have complemented improved surveillance, detection, and treatment of sepsis, but, despite these efforts, sepsis remains the most common cause of postoperative morbidity and mortality.[37–39] This observation is not a clinical failure but an observation that the microbiology and epidemiology of infectious complications after transplantation continue to change.

Understanding of the changing dynamics of infectious complications in ASORs must begin with the definition of an infectious complication that varies with allograft type. For liver and intestinal allografts, infectious complications after a technically successful surgical procedure represent allograft failure. This concept clarifies the important roles of each of these organs in immune function and pathogen protection. In pancreas and renal transplantation, immediate postoperative infectious complications may represent an iatrogenic event, an existing infection unappreciated at the time of surgery, or surgical complication.[40]

The changing landscape for microbiologic and viral infectious complications has evolved as a result of relaxing ASOR criteria with expansion of the donor pool.[41] The adoption of MELD as the liver allocation scheme fundamentally increased recipient acuity while donor selection criteria have been relaxed to ameliorate organ scarcity.[8] The functional mismatch created by high-acuity recipients, who have an increased requirement for immediate EAF, receiving transplanted allografts with limited immediate hepatic supply creates an opportunity for sepsis and multi–organ-system failure.[42]

In renal and pancreas transplantation, the widespread adoption of induction therapy with antilymphocyte antibody preparations in the immediate postoperative period provides an opportunity for pathogens secondary to abrupt impairment of cellular immunity. Avoiding volume overload, interstitial edema, and undesired areas of hemorrhage limit opportunities for infectious pathogens.

C difficile infection mandates particular attention because of its increasing incidence and morbidity.[43] *C difficile* infection occurs in approximately 19% of liver, 16% of kidney, 9% of intestinal, and 8% of pancreas-kidney recipients compared with less than 1% of patients without transplants.[44,45] *C difficile* may present as classic fulminant colitis with endotoxemic shock or more subtly as a manifestation of nonspecific symptoms including diarrhea.[45] For transplant recipients, the sequelae of diarrhea-induced hypotension, hypovolemia, and electrolyte disorders affect allograft function and predispose to thrombosis.[46] *C difficile* infections peak within 3 months following transplantation and result from antibiotic-induced floral changes, impaired immunity as a consequence of intense immunosuppression, and increased exposure to the health care setting.[47]

Various biomarkers including procalcitonin and C-reactive protein have been widely investigated in the setting of critically ill ASORs. To date, only an increasing C-reactive protein has been found to have clinical value in predicting an infectious event.[48,49]

Pulmonary Complications

Pulmonary complications can be infectious or noninfectious. Pulmonary infectious complications show variability according to allograft type. For renal and pancreas transplant recipients, pulmonary complications typically originate from an operative complication or the high incidence of diabetes, hypertension, coronary artery disease (CAD), and obstructive lung disease within these populations. The risk of aspiration on induction is high, particularly among pancreas recipients, who show diabetic gastroparesis.[28,50] In a multicenter study, the incidence of pneumonia among renal recipients admitted to the intensive care unit with acute respiratory failure was 35% with in-hospital mortality that exceeded 20%.[50] The physiology of cirrhosis is associated with restrictive lung disease secondary to ascites, hepatic hydrothorax, or obesity. Pretransplant hepatopulmonary syndrome persists in the immediate postoperative period and may require prolonged ventilation or oxygen administration. Acute respiratory distress syndrome resulting from bacterial translocation is the principal threat with small bowel transplantation.

Pneumonia is a leading cause of sepsis, prolonged posttransplant hospitalization, and mortality among ASORs. The incidence of hospital-acquired pneumonia within 7 days of liver transplantation approximates 15%.[38] The pathogens were 60% gram-negative and 40% gram-positive with greater than 90% sensitivity to broad-spectrum β-lactams and aminoglycosides. Multivariate analysis identified lactatemia, vasopressor requirements, Simplified Acute Physiology Score II (SAPSII) on admission, and mechanical ventilation exceeding 48 hours as being associated with development of pneumonia.[38] Early diagnostic bronchoscopy with short-term comprehensive empiric antibiotics decreases overall antibiotic exposure, reduces the potential for antibiotic resistance, and minimizes the morbidity associated with diagnostic delay.[51]

Noninfectious pulmonary complications include pleural effusion, atelectasis, diaphragmatic dysfunction, pneumothorax, pulmonary embolism, and pulmonary edema.[52] Pleural effusion, pneumothorax, and atelectasis are easily diagnosed and self-limited if treated early. Acute respiratory failure is common in liver and intestinal transplantation because of upper abdominal surgery, large intravascular volume shifts, and high transfusion requirements.[52] Acute respiratory failure among kidney and pancreas recipients is typically a complication of antilymphocyte globulin therapy.[53]

When evaluating pulmonary edema, it is essential to distinguish the hydrostatic versus permeability types. Hydrostatic pulmonary edema is common, particularly in liver transplant recipients, in which the incidence has been reported to exceed 50% in some series.[54] This process is self-limited and typically responds to diuretics with little impact on morbidity.

Permeability or noncardiogenic pulmonary edema portends a poor prognosis. Precipitating factors for this type of pulmonary edema include sepsis, gastric aspiration, and multiple transfusions.[55] In an observational analysis the cause of pulmonary edema was evaluated by comparing the protein content of pulmonary fluid with plasma protein content. Most liver recipients had noncardiogenic pulmonary edema, leading the investigators to conclude that the cause is transfusion-related acute lung injury (TRALI).[55]

The correlation of TRALI with posttransplant pulmonary edema supports the 2-event causal model. The initial priming event is a proinflammatory catalyst such as surgical stress or IRI that activates pulmonary endothelial cells and neutrophil sequestration within the pulmonary circulation. Antibodies, lipids, and biologic mediators from transfusion then sequentially activate these primed neutrophils to release a variety of molecules leading to endothelial cell damage, loss of capillary membrane integrity, capillary leak, and interstitial edema.[56]

Treatment of noncardiogenic pulmonary edema should incorporate lung protection strategies using low-tidal-volume ventilation.[57] Positive end-expiratory pressure has been discouraged secondary to theoretic concerns about reduction in venous return and impairment of hepatic venous outflow resulting in allograft congestion; however, emerging data in liver transplantation suggest that positive end-expiratory pressure of up to 15 cm H_2O does not affect Doppler flow velocities within the portal vein, hepatic artery, or hepatic veins.[58]

Cardiac Complications

Cardiovascular (CV) complications are a leading cause of morbidity and mortality, with the highest mortality observed in the immediate posttransplant period.[59–61] Although CV disease is highly prevalent among renal and pancreatic transplant candidates, increasing data refute the conventional concept of a cardioprotective effect of end-stage liver disease. Cirrhotics have a significantly higher prevalence of risk factors for obstructive CAD than the general population.[61,62] A consensus panel of the American Heart Association and American College of Cardiology has released guidelines for the evaluation and management of cardiac disease of kidney and liver transplant candidates.[63] The panel recognized an increased risk among ASORs for cardiac events but acknowledged the need for additional data to facilitate risk stratification.

Current data in liver transplantation suggest that preexisting CAD only contributes a limited component to posttransplant CV morbidity.[64] A notable exception is a subset of candidates with angiographically documented multivessel CAD, even in the absence of severe ($\geq$70%) coronary artery stenosis, which is associated with significantly increased mortality. Additional causes contributing to posttransplant CV morbidity include plaque instability, microvascular thrombosis secondary to transient hypercoagulable states, cirrhotic cardiomyopathy, and uremic cardiomyopathy. The lack of a correlation between obstructive CAD or revascularization before transplantation and CV morbidity has raised speculation that perioperative major adverse cardiac events are not caused by stable plaques propagating inward to create a stenosis, but by vulnerable plaque rupture or erosion that stimulates thrombus formation and arterial occlusion.

In renal transplant recipients, a single-center observational study determined no survival difference between candidates receiving coronary angiography (CA), coronary intervention, and no invasive cardiac intervention. These results imply that CAD screening may not be necessary and serve only to restrict access to a life-extending renal transplant.[65]

Early data on the sensitivity of cardiac biomarkers in identifying perioperative CV events is promising. In a retrospective study of liver recipients, pretransplant increase of serum troponin I was an independent risk factor for the occurrence of a posttransplant cardiac event.[66] A similar prospective study of kidney and kidney-pancreas recipients determined that pretransplant troponin I was a significant, independent predictor of CV mortality.[67]

Renal Complications

Renal failure following transplantation of a nonrenal organ is a common cause of morbidity and associated with a 4-fold increase in the relative risk of death.[17,68,69] In a landmark study, postoperative acute renal failure, defined as a 50% glomerular filtration rate reduction or requirement for renal replacement therapy (RRT), occurred in 7.6% of ASORs and doubled the risk of chronic renal failure.[17,69] Furthermore, ASORs have an estimated cumulative risk of developing end-stage renal disease that approaches 2% annually.[69] RRT after transplantation increases hospitalization, infectious complications, and mortality.[69] However, recent data suggest that any acute kidney injury (AKI), not just renal injury precipitating RRT, negatively affects long-term morbidity and mortality.[68,70] In a study of liver recipients, posttransplant creatinine changes of as little as 0.5 mg/dL significantly decreased patient and graft survival, with overall mortality corresponding with the severity of renal injury.[68]

Nephrotoxic immunosuppression and infectious prophylaxis compound the risk of AKI. The highest incidence of AKI is observed after intestinal transplantation because of surgical contributions, intense immunosuppression, and underlying allograft injury.[12] As long-term survival following intestinal transplantation increases, the effect of chronic kidney disease on survival has become apparent.[71]

The significance of posttransplant renal function has stimulated identification of biomarkers for earlier detection of perioperative renal injury. The 2 most studied markers are cystatin C and neutrophil gelatinase-associated lipocalin (NGAL). NGAL has shown the most promise through multiple prospective single-center studies of liver transplant recipients.[72–74] A study comparing NGAL with historical renal markers and intensive care unit organ failure scores showed that plasma NGAL was superior to creatinine at predicting AKI, particularly when combined with the APACHE (Acute Physiology and Chronic Health Evaluation) scoring system.[74] Cystatin C is a marker of renal function (not injury) and is independent of muscle mass, age, or sex. Cystatin C may reflect glomerular filtration fraction better than conventional serum markers such as creatinine.

Strategies to optimize posttransplant renal function have been widely disseminated. Modification of immunosuppression to include antibody induction therapy or addition of mycophenolate mofetil with calcineurin inhibitor sparing can be considered in addition to dose adjustment of prophylactic medications in patients with posttransplant AKI. Early detection of chronic calcineurin nephrotoxicity and conversion to renal-sparing immunosuppression is paramount to preserving renal function.

SUMMARY

The maturation of abdominal solid-organ transplantation as a clinical entity has brought new challenges to the intensivists caring for these patients. The relaxation of recipient criteria combined with expansion of the donor pool has opened the field to a wide spectrum of clinical situations. In this environment, donor factors, recipient comorbidities, intraoperative events, and estimation of EAF are essential. Recognition of EAF, optimization of the recipient in support of the allograft, and early treatment of postoperative complications provide a mechanism for serving the largest population of recipients with the widest variety of allografts.

REFERENCES

1. Perico N, Cattaneo D, Sayegh M, et al. Delayed graft function in kidney transplantation. Lancet 2004;364:1814–27.
2. Diaz G, O'Connor M. Cardiovascular and renal complications in patients receiving a solid-organ transplant. Curr Opin Crit Care 2011;17:382–9.
3. Squifflet J, Gruessner R, Sutherland D. The history of pancreas transplantation: past, present, and future. Acta Chir Belg 2008;108:367–78.
4. Ruiz P, Kato T, Tzakis A. Current status of transplantation of the small intestine. Transplantation 2007;83:1–6.
5. Scientific registry of transplant recipients. 2012 Annual data report. Available at: www.SRTR.org. Accessed May 1, 2013.
6. Port F, Bragg-Gresham J, Metzger R, et al. Donor characteristics associated with reduced graft survival: an approach to expanding the pool of kidney donors. Transplantation 2002;74:1281–6.
7. Alkofer B, Samstein B, Guarrera J, et al. Extended-donor criteria liver allografts. Semin Liver Dis 2006;26:221–33.
8. Busuttil R, Tanaka K. The utility of marginal donors in liver transplantation. Liver Transpl 2003;9:651–63.
9. Durand F, Renz J, Alkofer B, et al. Report of the Paris consensus meeting on expanded criteria donors in liver transplantation. Liver Transpl 2008;14: 1694–707.
10. Renz J, Kin C, Kinkhabwala M, et al. Utilization of extended donor criteria liver allografts maximizes donor use and patient access to liver transplantation. Ann Surg 2005;242:556–63.
11. Tector A, Mangus R, Chestovich P, et al. Use of extended criteria livers decreases wait time for liver transplantation without adversely impacting posttransplant survival. Ann Surg 2006;244:439–50.
12. Mangus R, Tector A, Kubal C, et al. Multivisceral transplantation: expanding indications and improving outcomes. J Gastrointest Surg 2013;17: 179–86.
13. Selck F, Grossman E, Ratner L, et al. Utilization, outcomes, and retransplantation of liver allografts from donation after cardiac death: implications for further expansion of the deceased-donor pool. Ann Surg 2008;248:599–607.
14. Renz J. Is DCD for liver transplantation DNR? Am J Transplant 2008;8:485–8.
15. Abt P, Desai N, Crawford M, et al. Survival following liver transplantation from non-heart-beating donors. Ann Surg 2004;239:87–92.
16. Ojo A, Wolfe R, Held P, et al. Delayed graft function: risk factors and implications for renal allograft survival. Transplantation 1997;63:968–74.
17. Ojo A, Held P, Port F, et al. Chronic renal failure after transplantation of a nonrenal organ. N Engl J Med 2003;349:931–40.

18. Singh R, Farney A, Rogers J, et al. Kidney transplantation from donation after cardiac death donors: lack of impact of delayed graft function on post-transplant outcomes. Clin Transplant 2011;25:255–64.
19. Locke J, Segev D, Warren D, et al. Outcomes of kidneys from donors after cardiac death: implications for allocation and preservation. Am J Transplant 2007;7: 1797–807.
20. Yarlagadda S, Coca S, Formica R, et al. Association between delayed graft function and allograft and patient survival: a systematic review and meta-analysis. Nephrol Dial Transplant 2009;24:1039–47.
21. Kamath P, Wiesner R, Malinchoc M, et al. A model to predict survival in patients with end-stage liver disease. Hepatology 2001;33:464–70.
22. Wiesner R, Lake J, Freeman R, et al. Model for end-stage liver disease (MELD) exception guidelines. Liver Transpl 2006;12:S85–7.
23. Olthoff K, Kulik L, Samstein B, et al. Validation of a current definition of early allograft dysfunction in liver transplant recipients and analysis of risk factors. Liver Transpl 2010;16:943–9.
24. Wagener G, Raffel B, Young AT, et al. Predicting early allograft failure and mortality after liver transplantation: the role of the postoperative model for end-stage liver disease score. Liver Transpl 2013;19(5):534–42.
25. Feng S, Goodrich N, Bragg-Gresham J, et al. Characteristics associated with liver graft failure: the concept of a donor risk index. Am J Transplant 2006;6:783–90.
26. Duffy J, Farmer D, Busuttil R. A quarter century of liver transplantation at UCLA. Clin Transplant 2007;165–70.
27. Barlow A, Hosgood S, Nicholson M. Current state of pancreas preservation and implications for DCD pancreas transplantation. Transplantation 2013;95(12): 1419–24.
28. Troppmann C. Complications after pancreas transplantation. Curr Opin Organ Transplant 2010;15:112–8.
29. Scalea J, Cooper M. Current concepts in the simultaneous transplantation of kidney and pancreas. J Intensive Care Med 2012;27:199–206.
30. Humar A, Kandaswamy R, Drangstveit M, et al. Prolonged preservation increases surgical complications after pancreas transplants. Surgery 2000;127:545–51.
31. Sharif A, Borrows R. Delayed graft function after kidney transplantation; the clinical perspective. Am J Kidney Dis 2013;62(1):150–8.
32. Small R, Shetzigovski I, Blachar A, et al. Redefining late acute graft pancreatitis: clinical presentation, radiologic findings, principles of management, and prognosis. Ann Surg 2008;247:1058–63.
33. Troppmann C. Surgical complications. In: Gruessner R, Sutherland D, editors. Pancreas transplantation. New York: Springer; 2004. p. 206–37.
34. Gimenez J, Bluth E, Simon A, et al. Evaluation of pancreatic allografts with sonography. J Ultrasound Med 2012;31:1041–51.
35. Fishbein T, Kaufman S, Florman S, et al. Isolated intestinal transplantation: proof of clinical efficacy. Transplantation 2003;76:636–40.
36. Razonable R, Findlay J, O'Riordan A, et al. Critical care issues in patients after liver transplantation. Liver Transpl 2011;17:511–27.
37. Paugam-Burtz C, Albuquerque M, Baron G, et al. Plasma proteome to look for diagnostic biomarkers of early bacterial sepsis after liver transplantation. Anesthesiology 2010;112:926–35.
38. Weiss E, Dahmani S, Bert F, et al. Early-onset pneumonia after liver transplantation: microbiological findings and therapeutic consequences. Liver Transpl 2010;16:1178–85.

39. Karvellas C, McPhail M, Pink F, et al. Bloodstream infection after elective liver transplantation is associated with increased mortality in patients with cirrhosis. J Crit Care 2011;26:468–74.

40. Fishman J. Infections in immunocompromised hosts and organ transplant recipients: essentials. Liver Transpl 2011;17:S34–7.

41. Fishman J. Infection in solid-organ transplant recipients. N Engl J Med 2007; 357:2601–14.

42. Renz J. A critical analysis of liver allograft utilization from the US deceased donor pool. Liver Transpl 2010;16:543–7.

43. Dubberke E, Burdette S. AST infectious diseases community of practice. Clostridium difficile infections in solid organ transplantation. Am J Transplant 2013; 13:42–9.

44. Dubberke E, Butler A, Yokoe D, et al. Multicenter study of Clostridium difficile infection rates from 2000 to 2006. Infect Control Hosp Epidemiol 2010;31: 1030–7.

45. Boutros M, Al-Shaibi M, Chan G, et al. Clostridium difficile colitis: increasing incidence, risk factors, and outcomes in solid organ transplant recipients. Transplantation 2012;93:1051–7.

46. Dallal R, Harbrecht B, Boujoukas A, et al. Fulminant Clostridium difficile: an under appreciated and increasing cause of death and complications. Ann Surg 2002;235:363–72.

47. Riddle D, Dubberke E. Clostridium difficile infection in solid organ transplant recipients. Curr Opin Organ Transplant 2008;13:592–600.

48. van den Broek M, Olde Damink S, Winkens B, et al. Procalcitonin as a prognostic marker for infectious complications in liver transplant recipient in an intensive care unit. Liver Transpl 2010;16:402–10.

49. Zazula R, Prucha M, Tyll T, et al. Induction of procalcitonin in liver transplant patients treated with anti-thymocyte globulin. Crit Care 2007;11(6): R131.

50. Canet E, Osman D, Lambert J, et al. Acute respiratory failure in kidney transplant recipients: a multicenter study. Crit Care 2011;15(2):R91.

51. Harris B, Lowy F, Stover D, et al. Diagnostic bronchoscopy in solid-organ and hematopoietic stem cell transplantation. Ann Am Thorac Soc 2013;10:39–49.

52. Kotloff R. Noninfectious pulmonary complications of liver, heart, and kidney transplantation. Clin Chest Med 2005;26:623–9.

53. Shorr A, Abbott K, Agadoa L. Acute respiratory distress syndrome after kidney transplantation: epidemiology, risk factors, and outcomes. Crit Care Med 2003; 31:1325–30.

54. Snowden C, Hughes T, Rose J, et al. Pulmonary edema in patients after liver transplantation. Liver Transpl 2000;6:466–70.

55. Yost C, Matthay M, Gropper M. Etiology of acute pulmonary edema during liver transplantation. Chest 2001;119:219–23.

56. Silliman C. The two-event model of transfusion-related acute lung injury. Crit Care Med 2006;34:S124–31.

57. Acute Respiratory Distress Syndrome Network. Ventilation with lower tidal volumes as compared with traditional tidal volumes for acute lung injury and the acute respiratory distress syndrome. N Engl J Med 2000;342:1301–8.

58. Saner F, Olde Damink S, Pavlakovic G, et al. How far can we go with positive end-expiratory pressure (PEEP) in liver transplant patients? J Clin Anesth 2010;22:104–9.

59. Lin K, Stewart D, Cooper S, et al. Pre-transplant cardiac testing for kidney-pancreas transplant candidates and association with cardiac outcomes. Clin Transplant 2001;15:269–75.
60. United States Renal Data System. 2011 annual data report. Bethesda (MD): National Institutes of Health, National Institute of Diabetes and Digestive and Kidney Diseases; 2011. Available at: www.usrds.org. Accessed May 01, 2013.
61. Findlay J, Wen D, Mandell M. Cardiac risk evaluation for abdominal transplantation. Curr Opin Organ Transplant 2010;15:363–7.
62. Tiukinhoy-Laing S, Rossi J, Bayram M, et al. Cardiac hemodynamic and coronary angiographic characteristics of patients being evaluated for liver transplantation. Am J Cardiol 2006;98:178–81.
63. Lentine K, Cost S, Weir M, et al. Cardiac disease evaluation and management among kidney and liver transplantation candidates. J Am Coll Cardiol 2012; 60:434–80.
64. Little W, Applegate R. The shadows leave a doubt – The angiographic recognition of vulnerable coronary artery plaques. J Am Coll Cardiol 1999;33: 1362–4.
65. Patel R, Mark P, Johnston N, et al. Prognostic value of cardiovascular screening in potential renal transplant recipients: a single-center prospective observational study. Am J Transplant 2008;8:1673–83.
66. Coss E, Watt K, Pedersen R, et al. Predictors of cardiovascular events after liver transplantation: a role for pretransplant serum troponin levels. Liver Transpl 2011;17:23–31.
67. Claes K, Bammens B, Evenepoel P, et al. Troponin I is a predictor of acute cardiac events in the immediate postoperative renal transplant period. Transplantation 2010;89:341–6.
68. Barri Y, Sanchez E, Jennings L, et al. Acute kidney injury following liver transplantation: definition and outcome. Liver Transpl 2009;15:475–83.
69. Ojo A. Renal disease in recipients of nonrenal solid organ transplantation. Semin Nephrol 2007;27:498–507.
70. Zhu M, Li Y, Xia Q, et al. Strong impact of acute kidney injury on survival after liver transplantation. Transplant Proc 2010;42:3634–8.
71. Mujtaba S, Sharfuddin A, Yaqub M, et al. Risk factors for native kidney dysfunction in patients with abdominal multivisceral/small bowel transplantation. Clin Transplant 2012;26:E351–8.
72. Wagener G, Minhaz M, Matis FA, et al. Urinary neutrophil gelatinase-associated lipocalin as a marker of acute kidney injury after orthotopic liver transplantation. Liver Transpl 2011;26(5):1717–23.
73. Niemann C, Walia A, Waldman J, et al. Acute kidney injury during liver transplantation as determined by neutrophil gelatinase-associated lipocalin. Liver Transpl 2009;15:1852–60.
74. Portal A, McPhail M, Bruce M, et al. Neutrophil gelatinase-associated lipocalin predicts acute kidney injury in patients undergoing liver transplantation. Liver Transpl 2010;16:1257–66.

Current Research on Organ Donor Management

Mitchell Sally, MD, Darren Malinoski, MD*

KEYWORDS

- Organ donor management • Organ donation • Graft outcomes • Transplantation
- Donor management goals

KEY POINTS

- A shortage of organs is available for transplantation, and therefore improving the critical care provided to potential donors may increase the quantity and quality of the organs.
- A brief summary of the existing organ donor management literature is discussed and descriptions of ongoing studies are presented.
- Standardizing donor management practices through the use of bundles/checklists has the potential to improve outcomes and provide a framework for future, randomized studies.

INTRODUCTION

A shortage of organs is available for transplantation, with 116,000 patients on the Organ Procurement and Transplantation Network/United Network for Organ Sharing (UNOS) wait list.[1] Because the demand for organs outweighs the supply, considerable care must be taken to maximize the number of organs transplanted per donor and optimize the quality of the organs recovered.

Studies designed to determine optimal donor management therapies are limited, and this research has many challenges.[2] Although evidenced-based guidelines for managing potential organ donors do not exist, research in this area is increasing. This article reviews the existing literature and highlights some recent trials that can guide management.

Neurologic death is accompanied by myriad immunologic, hemodynamic, and endocrine abnormalities.[3] This article focuses on management of the cardiovascular, pulmonary, renal, hepatic, pancreatic, endocrine, and coagulation organ systems in potential donors after neurologic determination of death (DNDDs) in the intensive care unit (ICU) and the operating room.

Portland VA Medical Center, Oregon Health & Science University, PO Box 1034/Mail Code P3ANES, Portland, OR 97207, USA
* Corresponding author.
E-mail address: malinosk@ohsu.edu

Anesthesiology Clin 31 (2013) 737–748
http://dx.doi.org/10.1016/j.anclin.2013.08.004
1932-2275/13/$ – see front matter Published by Elsevier Inc.
anesthesiology.theclinics.com

CARDIOVASCULAR SYSTEM

Up to 34% of potential DNDDs can experience cardiovascular collapse, and aggressive critical care management is needed to avoid the loss of organs from these donors.[4] Echocardiography is routinely used to assess the left ventricular function of a potential donor heart. Cardiac catheterization may be more selectively used for donors older than 55 years and younger patients with a history of cocaine use, or those with 3 or more risk factors for coronary artery disease, such as hypertension, diabetes, dyslipidemia, prolonged smoking history, or family history of premature coronary artery disease.[5]

In the setting of left ventricular dysfunction, pulmonary artery catheter-directed management can maximize donor recovery. Properly managed younger hearts with left ventricular dysfunction have been shown to markedly recover function after transplantation.[6] At minimum, all DNDDs should have either central venous pressure (CVP) guidance or other fluid responsiveness monitors for resuscitation and support. If a pulmonary artery catheter is used, it is designed to optimize cardiac output and maintain normal preload and afterload. The role of adjunctive hormone therapy to improve cardiac function is discussed later.

In up to 90% of donors, endogenous vasopressin is noted to be either absent or low[7] and, in donors requiring catecholamine support, is often inadequate to maintain homeostasis.[8] In a retrospective study by Plurad and colleagues,[9] the use of arginine vasopressin in the DNDD was associated with more organs transplanted per donor. Additional agents, such as dopamine, phenylephrine, or norepinephrine, may be titrated as needed to maximize end-organ perfusion.

Echocardiogram changes and cardiac arrhythmias are common in DNDDs and are thought to be caused by both metabolic and electrolyte abnormalities and infarction of the conduction system. The use of standard antiarrhythmic therapy is appropriate. An important caveat is that vagus nerve disruption in the brain stem may result in a bradyarrhythmia, which is resistant to the effects of atropine, and therefore a β-adrenergic agonist, such as isoproterenol or epinephrine, may be required.[10] Untreated arrhythmias may become completely refractory to management if not treated early and aggressively.

PULMONARY SYSTEM

Standard criteria for lung donation stipulate that suitable donors must have a ratio of Pao_2 to fraction of inspired oxygen (Fio_2) greater than 300 mm Hg (Pao_2 >300 mm Hg with 100% Fio_2 on 5 cm H_2O positive end-expiratory pressure [PEEP]). The origins of this threshold are unclear and likely based on conjecture rather than observation. Although most centers follow this guideline in selecting donors, limited but conflicting experience with donors who deviate from this standard has occurred. In a multicenter French retrospective review of transplants performed between 1988 and 1998, donor Pao_2:Fio_2 less than 350 mm Hg was associated with a steep increase in the risk of death.[11] In contrast, Luckraz and colleagues[12] retrospectively reviewed 362 donor and recipient pairs over a 17-year period and found no difference in 1- and 5-year survivals for recipients with donor Pao_2:Fio_2 less than 300 mm Hg compared with greater than 300 mm Hg. Reyes and colleagues[13] analyzed the UNOS database containing more than 10,000 primary transplants in the United States and found that donor Pao_2:Fio_2 was less than 300 mm Hg in 18% of cases (n = 1751 recipients), and survival to 7 years for this group was similar to that of recipients in whom donor Pao_2:Fio_2 exceeded 300 mm Hg.

Tailored lung donor management protocols involving diuresis, therapeutic bronchoscopy, chest physiotherapy, and lung recruitment maneuvers have been shown to improve oxygenation parameters in donors who initially fail to meet the standard oxygenation requirement. In a study from Australia, an aggressive lung donor protocol led to achievement of a $Pao_2:Fio_2$ greater than 300 mm Hg in 20 of 59 potential donors whose initial oxygenation was less than this threshold.[14] A similar strategy, including use of a recruitment maneuver of pressure-controlled ventilation at an inspiratory pressure of 25 cm H_2O and PEEP of 15 cm H_2O for 2 hours, was used by the San Antonio lung transplant program. Of 98 donors, one-third converted from unacceptable to acceptable $Pao_2:Fio_2$ ratios in response to this protocol.[15]

Traditionally, donor management protocols used by organ procurement organizations (OPOs) recommend using tidal volumes of 10 to 15 mL/kg when ventilating potential lung donors. A recent multicenter randomized trial examined a lung-protective ventilatory strategy similar to that used in patients with acute respiratory distress syndrome.[16] Potential donors were randomized to 1 of 2 strategies: a conventional protocol using tidal volumes of 10 to 12 mL/kg, 3 to 5 cm PEEP, and an open circuit for both suctioning and apnea tests; or a lung-protective protocol using tidal volumes of 6 to 8 mL/kg, 8 to 10 cm PEEP, a closed circuit for suctioning, continuous positive airway pressure equal to previous PEEP for apnea tests, and recruitment maneuvers after any disconnection from the ventilator. Use of the lung-protective protocol doubled lung recovery rates (54% vs 27%; $P<.005$) compared with the conventional ventilator protocol, but the relative benefits of each protective strategy are unknown.

A smaller, single-center retrospective study of 45 potential lung donors compared lung transplantation rates when a standard, assist-control ventilatory mode was used versus when airway pressure release ventilation (APRV) was used.[17] Donors managed with APRV had a significantly higher rate of successful lung recovery (84% vs 18%) and similar graft survival rates compared with the conventionally ventilated group and national averages.

Bronchoscopy allows an easy and quick visual assessment of the airway anatomy and has been shown to add to noninvasive assessments. Riou and colleagues[18] reported that bronchoscopy was abnormal in 10 of 26 (38%) potential organ donors with normal radiographs and Pao_2 greater than 400 mm Hg. The most common bronchoscopic abnormalities reported included aspirated gastric contents or blood, and purulent secretions.[17] Most centers deem the presence of aspirated gastric contents or purulent secretions that fail to clear with suctioning as a contraindication to lung donation. Bronchoscopy can also clear mucous plugs or blood clots that may contribute to impaired oxygenation.

Limited data are available on lung procurement and recipient outcomes with regard to different fluid management protocols. However, studies in patients with acute respiratory distress syndrome provide some insight. One large prospective trial randomized these patients to either a liberal fluid management strategy (target CVP, 10–14 mm Hg or pulmonary artery occlusion pressure [PAOP], 14–18 mm) or a conservative strategy (target CVP, <4 mm Hg and PAOP, <8 mm Hg).[18] The conservative fluid strategy was associated with superior oxygenation and a decrease in duration of mechanical ventilation and need for intensive care, and no increase in other organ failure (eg, renal, hepatic).

The best evidence supporting a conservative fluid management strategy in potential lung donors comes from the San Antonio lung transplant group.[15] As part of a lung donor–specific management protocol, they incorporated a conservative fluid management strategy that minimized use of crystalloids and used diuretics to maintain neutral or negative fluid balance. Their protocol was associated with increased lung procurement without affecting other organs for transplantation, but the degree to which this was from conservative fluid management as opposed to other components of their protocol (eg, recruitment maneuvers) cannot be determined. Results of a study of 404 kidney recipients provide assurance that a conservative fluid strategy with CVP of 6 mm Hg or less does not adversely affect renal graft survival nor increase the risk of delayed graft function.[10] This finding argues against the widely held notion that fluid strategies to optimize lung and kidney donation are in direct conflict.

ENDOCRINE SYSTEM

Ischemia of the hypothalamic-pituitary axis during neurologic death can lead to diminished circulating levels of adrenocorticotropic hormone, thyroid stimulating hormone, and vasopressin, resulting in important endocrine derangements with marked systemic effects. Additionally, the stress response to neurologic death causes the activation of leukocytes and a pronounced inflammatory response.

Vasopressin

Vasopressin (or antidiuretic hormone) acts on its V1 subtype receptor found in vascular smooth muscle (vasopressor activity) and the V2 subtype found in renal collecting duct epithelia, which increases water permeability (antidiuretic activity). Up to 90% of DNDDs are noted to have a severe deficiency in vasopressin, which contributes to the cardiovascular collapse and resultant hypotension.[8,19] In addition, neurogenic diabetes insipidus (DI) is present in nearly half of all DNDDs.[4] When uncontrolled, this condition can result in a massive hypoosmolar diuresis and electrolyte abnormalities, most commonly hypernatremia.

The correction of DI and fluid status is of paramount importance to preserve perfusion. Volume resuscitation with isotonic fluids is necessary to correct hypovolemia, and then hypotonic fluids can be used to correct the hypernatremia that will likely remain. In the setting of persistent hypotension despite adequate volume replacement, arginine vasopressin can be used to treat both the vasodilatory shock and the DI. In DNDDs who do not require vasopressor support, 1-desamino-8-D-arginine vasopressin is highly selective for the V2 subtype alone, and may be used as an adjunctive treatment for DI.

Thyroxine

Diminished circulating levels of thyroid hormone (T3/T4) have been implicated as one of the reasons for hemodynamic instability and metabolic acidosis in DNDDs.[3,20–23] Therapeutic replacement with T3 has been associated with reversal of anaerobic metabolism and subsequent stabilization of cardiac function,[21,24] reductions in inotropic support, and decreases in donors lost from cardiac instability.[25–29] T4 administration has also been associated with significantly more organs procured per donor (3.9 ± 1.7 vs 3.2 ± 1.7; $P = .048$).[30]

Glucose abnormalities may be severe in DNDDs. After development of neurologic death, insulin levels can decrease up to 50% of baseline at 3 hours, and even further to 20% of baseline at 13 hours.[23] The resulting pronounced hyperglycemia has many potentially harmful effects, and leads to increased risk of allograft dysfunction. Uncontrolled glucose levels promote tissue damage through protein glycosylation, and this is especially true in the renal system. Additionally, osmotic diuresis resulting from glucose spillage may overwhelm renal medullary function, and contribute to the diuresis already initiated in neurologic death. Lastly, hyperglycemia results in oxidative damage and a proinflammatory state.[31,32]

Increased glucose levels in the DNDD correlate with higher serum creatinine levels before organ recovery,[33] and recent unpublished data from Sally and colleagues

(2014, in press) UNOS Region 5 (Southwestern United States) suggest that maintaining glucose levels of 180 mg/dL or less is associated with both increased organs transplanted per donor and improved graft outcomes.

Steroids

The body experiences a massive inflammatory response after brain death, characterized by elevations in circulating cytokines such as interleukin-6 and tumor necrosis factor.[34] This cytokine surge can be detrimental to the function and survival of transplanted organs,[35] with increased plasma levels of interleukin-6 being associated with decreased liver graft survival.[36] Animal studies have shown neurologic death upregulating intercellular adhesion molecule-1 expression and leukocyte infiltration into peripheral organs, and a time-dependent progression of immune-mediated organ dysfunction.[37] Steroids combat this inflammatory cascade through decreasing levels of serum cytokines,[38] resulting in improved posttransplant organ viability.[39] Corticosteroids also act to overcome the relative adrenal insufficiency resulting from the stress of traumatic brain injury and, ultimately, neurologic death.[7,40,41]

RENAL SYSTEM

The systemic inflammatory response, sympathetic storm, and subsequent cardiovascular collapse that follow neurologic death all have deleterious effects on the renal system. Although dopamine administration is no longer recommended as a first-line vasopressor in the management of the DNDD because of its tachycardic and proarrhythmic effects, transplanted kidneys that come from donors treated with low-dose dopamine have been shown to have better initial graft function in their recipients. Specifically, recipients have been shown to require a shorter duration of hemodialysis after transplantation.[42] It is thought that preconditioning of the transplanted organs with dopamine may make them better able to withstand ischemic damage during cold preservation.[43] Maintaining adequate perfusion and controlling hyperglycemia are also critical to supporting the renal system of potential organ donors, and these strategies were discussed previously. In terms of the type of fluid to be used for resuscitation, isotonic crystalloids are generally preferred, with blood products and colloids being reserved for specific circumstances. Albumin 5% and hydroxyethyl starch (HES) are commonly available colloid solutions. However, HES use is associated with acute kidney injury and coagulopathy in critically ill patients.[44,45] The only prospective randomized controlled trial examining the use of colloids during donor management involved 27 donors and compared a standardized resuscitation strategy with gelatin plus large-molecular-weight HES (200 kDa) versus gelatin alone.[46] Delayed renal graft function was significantly higher in the HES group (33% vs 5%), as was the average 10-day recipient serum creatinine level. Taken together, these data do not support the use of HES in potential organ donors.

HEPATIC SYSTEM

Hypernatremia has been the most widely studied donor condition in regard to hepatic outcomes after transplantation. Several studies have suggested that donor plasma sodium greater than 155 mEq/dL is damaging to the liver,[24,47] although more recent studies have refuted this finding.[48] It is theorized that donor hypernatremia promotes the influx of osmotic molecules into hepatocytes after transplantation into a recipient with normal sodium levels, and the subsequent water influx promotes cell lysis. Although cellular dysfunction is clearly observed,[37,49,50] perhaps because of its tremendous metabolic reserve, the liver as a whole seems more tolerant to the dramatic changes that occur around the time of neurologic death compared with other solid organs.[51]

PANCREAS

To date, a comprehensive analysis regarding donor management and pancreas outcomes is lacking. An early study showed that donor hyperglycemia and immunologic variables are risk factors for pancreas graft loss.[52] The evaluation of other factors, such as insulin management, glycemic thresholds, and overall donor management, has not been specifically applied to pancreas grafts, and provide ripe areas for further research.

COAGULATION AND THERMOREGULATION DISORDERS

Hypothermia and acidosis, along with the dilution of clotting factors, fibrinogen, and platelets, can contribute to a state of disseminated intravascular coagulation and uncontrollable bleeding.[53] Massive transfusion protocols including the use of fresh frozen plasma, platelets, and cryoprecipitate are often required. Recent consensus recommended transfusion of packed red blood cells to a hematocrit greater than 30% for organ donors to maximize end-organ oxygen delivery, but data supporting this practice are limited.[5] However, spontaneous hypothermia from dysregulation and shock may be associated with different physiologic effects than induced therapeutic hypothermia, and studies are currently underway to prospectively assess both the impact of mild hypothermia induced for life-saving purposes before neurologic death as well as for organ-preserving purposes after authorization for donation.

DONOR MANAGEMENT GOALS

Approximately 90% of all organ donors become candidates after a neurologic determination of death. Before this, these potential donors are initially managed with the goal of optimizing brain tissue perfusion and clinical outcomes. After the declaration of neurologic death, however, the treating intensivist must focus on maximizing the well-being of as many other organs as possible, thus preserving the option of organ donation for the patient and their family. Similar to other critically ill patients, the treatments needed to optimize the physiologic state of a particular organ might be contrary to the interests of another. Unless the intensivist, anesthesiologist, and OPO coordinator know a priori that a particular organ will not be suitable for transplantation, they are faced with a delicate balancing act between the competing needs of several different organ systems.

One area of controversy surrounds the optimal fluid resuscitation strategy in a multiple-organ donor, with the potential for opposing goals between lungs and other organs. In general, aggressive fluid resuscitation is recommended to maintain a CVP of 8 to 12 mm Hg and a systolic arterial pressure between 90 and 140 mm Hg to stabilize the hemodynamic derangements that occur in most DNDDs and maintain perfusion of all of the organ systems.[54] However, in lung donors, it has been shown that maintenance of a CVP between 8 and 10 mm Hg may result in an increased alveolar arterial oxygen gradient when compared with potential donors maintained between 4 and 6 mm Hg, putting hydration of the kidneys and other viscera in conflict with optimization of the lungs.[19] Contrary to this report, several studies have shown that general optimization of cardiac function and volume status in DNDDs improves the viability of other transplantable organs.[55–58]

In a retrospective study of 308 donors, Abdelnour and Pieke[57] showed that in donors who received hormone replacement therapy, a CVP less than 10 mm Hg was associated with more hearts, lungs, and kidneys transplanted. Similarly, in a study by Minambres and colleagues,[56] a negative or even fluid balance with a CVP of 6 mm Hg or less was not associated with worse renal graft outcomes. In a prospective study comparing rates of renal delayed graft function in multiorgan donors, the use of cardiac or pancreas grafts was associated with lower rates, whereas the use of lungs from the same donor did not affect outcomes.[58]

To balance the critical care provided to support multiple organ systems, multiple groups have established sets of standardized critical care end points to guide the bedside management of potential organ donors.[10,58–62] Many OPOs have created checklists, or bundles, of these end points and termed them *donor management goals* (DMGs). The current DMGs used in UNOS Region 5 aim to balance the interests of all organ systems and are shown in **Table 1**. Several groups have found that more organs are transplanted per donor when DMGs are met by the OPO before organ recovery.[59–62] In addition, recent work in Region 5 has also shown that having these critical care end points achieved in the donor hospital ICU, before authorization for donation, is associated with more organs transplanted per donor and less delayed graft function in the recipients of kidneys from these donors.[58,59]

CONSIDERATIONS DURING ORGAN RECOVERY

Once an organ donor has been successfully managed in the ICU and organs have been allocated for recovery and transplantation, care of the donor shifts to the anesthesiologist in the operating room. The goals of management remain the maintenance of hemodynamic stability and other physiologic parameters/DMGs, and a few unique practices during the surgical recovery process are worthy of discussion.

Chemical neuromuscular paralysis is frequently administered to block muscle twitching caused by spinal reflexes to painful stimuli. Positive hemodynamic responses to stimuli are also still present in the DNDD, and may include spinal reflexes or reflex arc–mediated adrenal medullary stimulation.[63,64] Prostaglandins may be administered for lung-protective effects and can cause a profound hypotension, for which the anesthesiologist must be prepared. Additionally, around the time of aortic

Table 1
UNOS Region 5 donor management goals

Donor Management Goals	Parameters
Mean arterial pressure	60–110 mm Hg
Central venous pressure	4–12 mm Hg
Ejection fraction	$\geq$50%
Vasopressors	$\leq$1 and low dose[a]
Arterial blood gas pH	7.3–7.5
$Pao_2{:}Fio_2$	$\geq$300
Serum sodium	$\leq$155 mEq/L
Blood glucose	$\leq$180 mg/dL
Urine output	$\geq$0.5 mL/kg/h over 4 h

[a] Low dose of vasopressors is defined as: dopamine $\leq$10 µg/kg/min, phenylephrine $\leq$1 µg/kg/min, or norepinephrine $\leq$0.2 µg/kg/min.

cross-clamping, mannitol and Lasix are often administered to protect renal function, and the resulting diuresis may also promote hypotension.

After aortic cross-clamping, the role of the anesthesiologist is generally limited. The exception is in the case of lung recovery, which requires the lungs to be manually ventilated until removal. Care must be taken to avoid overinflating the lungs, causing additional barotrauma.

Lastly, the operating room can become the site in which many procurement professionals are working simultaneously and expeditiously in tight quarters. Effective communication among all providers, and the establishment of an overall leader directing the process as a whole, make the procurement proceed optimally.

SUMMARY AND FUTURE DIRECTIONS

Careful management of the potential donor, both before and after neurologic death, is crucial for successful outcomes of organ transplantation. Many studies have shown that adherence to DMGs is associated with improved outcomes, and these should be used as guides in optimizing the physiology of all the organ systems. However, despite vast improvements in donor management over the past decades, further research is needed. Recent studies examining topics such as using preload responsiveness to guide fluid resuscitation,[65] N-acetylcysteine,[66] and the use of vasopressin[9] have focused on testable hypotheses and opened the door for future studies. A recent editorial describes an urgent need for prospective, randomized trials involving deceased organ donors, citing organ donation as having a paucity of current clinical trials.[67] The hope is that this call for action will lead to further advances in the field of organ donor management. Critical care providers, inside the ICU and the operating room, are poised to have a significant influence in these efforts.

REFERENCES

1. Annual report of the U.S. Organ procurement and transplantation network and the scientific registry of transplant recipients: transplant data 1994–2013. Department of Health and Human Services, Health Resources and Services Administration, Healthcare Systems Bureau, Division of Transplantation, Rockville, MD; United Network for Organ Sharing, Richmond, VA. Ann Arbor (MI): University Renal Research and Education Association; 2013.
2. Abt PL, Marsh CL, Dunn TB, et al. Challenges to research and innovation to optimize deceased donor organ quality and quantity. Am J Transplant 2013;13: 1400–4.
3. Novitzky D, Cooper DK, Morrell D, et al. Change from aerobic to anaerobic metabolism after brain death, and reversal following triiodothyronine therapy. Transplantation 1988;45:32–6.
4. Salim A, Martin M, Brown C, et al. Complications of brain death: frequency and impact on organ retrieval. Am Surg 2006;72:377–81.
5. Zaroff JG, Rosengard BR, Armstrong WF, et al. Consensus conference report: maximizing use of organs recovered from the cadaver donor: cardiac recommendations, March 28-29, 2001, Crystal City, Va. Circulation 2002;106:836–41.
6. Milano A, Livi U, Casula R, et al. Influence of marginal donors on early results after heart transplantation. Transplant Proc 1993;25:3158–9.
7. Howlett TA, Keogh AM, Perry L, et al. Anterior and posterior pituitary function in brain-stem-dead donors. A possible role for hormonal replacement therapy. Transplantation 1989;47:828–34.

8. Chen JM, Cullinane S, Spanier TB, et al. Vasopressin deficiency and pressor hypersensitivity in hemodynamically unstable organ donors. Circulation 1999;100: II244–6.

9. Plurad DS, Bricker S, Neville A, et al. Arginine vasopressin significantly increases the rate of successful organ procurement in potential donors. Am J Surg 2012;204:856–61.

10. Wood KE, Becker BN, McCartney JG, et al. Care of the potential organ donor. N Engl J Med 2004;351:2730–9.

11. Thabut G, Mal H, Cerrina J, et al. Influence of donor characteristics on outcome after lung transplantation: a multicenter study. J Heart Lung Transplant 2005;24: 1347–53.

12. Luckraz H, White P, Sharples LD, et al. Short- and long-term outcomes of using pulmonary allograft donors with low PO2. J Heart Lung Transplant 2005;24: 470–3.

13. Reyes KG, Mason DP, Thulta L, et al. Guidelines for donor lung selection: time for revision? Ann Thorac Surg 2010;89:1756–64.

14. Gabbay E, Williams TJ, Griffiths AP, et al. Maximizing the utilization of donor organs offered for lung transplantation. Am J Respir Crit Care Med 1999;160:265–71.

15. Angel LF, Levine DJ, Restrepo MI, et al. Impact of a lung transplantation donor-management protocol on lung donation and recipient outcomes. Am J Respir Crit Care Med 2006;174:710–6.

16. Mascia L, Pasero D, Slutsky AS, et al. Effect of a lung protective strategy for organ donors on eligibility and availability of lungs for transplantation: a randomized controlled trial. JAMA 2010;304:2620–7.

17. Hanna K, Seder CW, Weinberger JB, et al. Airway pressure release ventilation and successful lung donation. Arch Surg 2011;146:325–8.

18. Riou B, Guesede R, Jacquens Y, et al. Fiberoptic bronchoscopy in brain-dead organ donors. Am J Respir Crit Care Med 1994;150:558–60.

19. Pennefather SH, Bullock RE, Mantle D, et al. Use of low dose arginine vasopressin to support brain-dead organ donors. Transplantation 1995;59:58–62.

20. Salter DR, Dyke CM, Wechsler AS. Triiodothyronine (T3) and cardiovascular therapeutics: a review. J Card Surg 1992;7:363–74.

21. Novitzky D, Cooper DK, Reichart B. Value of triiodothyronine (T3) therapy to brain-dead potential organ donors. J Heart Transplant 1986;5:486–7.

22. Novitzky D, Cooper DK, Reichart B. Hemodynamic and metabolic responses to hormonal therapy in brain-dead potential organ donors. Transplantation 1987; 43:852–4.

23. Wicomb WN, Cooper DK, Novitzky D. Impairment of renal slice function following brain death, with reversibility of injury by hormonal therapy. Transplantation 1986;41:29–33.

24. Gonzalez FX, Rimola A, Grande L, et al. Predictive factors of early postoperative graft function in human liver transplantation. Hepatology 1994;20:565–73.

25. Cooper DK, Novitzky D, Wicomb WN. The pathophysiological effects of brain death on potential donor organs, with particular reference to the heart. Ann R Coll Surg Engl 1989;71:261–6.

26. Zuppa AF, Nadkarni V, Davis L, et al. The effect of a thyroid hormone infusion on vasopressor support in critically ill children with cessation of neurologic function. Crit Care Med 2004;32:2318–22.

27. Novitzky D, Cooper DK, Chaffin JS, et al. Improved cardiac allograft function following triiodothyronine therapy to both donor and recipient. Transplantation 1990;49:311–6.

28. Novitzky D. Novel actions of thyroid hormone: the role of triiodothyronine in cardiac transplantation. Thyroid 1996;6:531–6.
29. Salim A, Vassiliu P, Velmahos GC, et al. The role of thyroid hormone administration in potential organ donors. Arch Surg 2001;136:1377–80.
30. Salim A, Martin M, Brown C, et al. Using thyroid hormone in brain-dead donors to maximize the number of organs available for transplantation. Clin Transplant 2007;21:405–9.
31. Fahy BG, Sheehy AM, Coursin DB. Glucose control in the intensive care unit. Crit Care Med 2009;37:1769–76.
32. Marik PE, Raghavan M. Stress-hyperglycemia, insulin and immunomodulation in sepsis. Intensive Care Med 2004;30:748–56.
33. Blasi-ibanez A, Hirose R, Feiner J, et al. Predictors associated with terminal renal function in deceased organ donors in the intensive care unit. Anesthesiology 2009;110:333–41.
34. Pratschke J, Wilhelm MJ, Kusaka M, et al. Accelerated rejection of renal allografts from brain-dead donors. Ann Surg 2000;232:263–71.
35. Deng MC, Erren M, Kammerling L, et al. The relation of interleukin-6, tumor necrosis factor-alpha, IL-2, and IL-2 receptor levels to cellular rejection, allograft dysfunction, and clinical events early after cardiac transplantation. Transplantation 1995;60:1118–24.
36. Murugan R, Venkataraman R, Wahed AS, et al. Increased plasma interleukin-6 in donors is associated with lower recipient hospital-free survival after cadaveric organ transplantation. Crit Care Med 2008;36:1810–6.
37. van Der Hoeven JA, Ter horst GJ, Molema G, et al. Effects of brain death and hemodynamic status on function and immunologic activation of the potential donor liver in the rat. Ann Surg 2000;232:804–13.
38. Kuecuek O, Mantouvalou L, Klemz R, et al. Significant reduction of proinflammatory cytokines by treatment of the brain-dead donor. Transplant Proc 2005;37:387–8.
39. Kotsch K, Ulrich F, Reutzel-selke A, et al. Methylprednisolone therapy in deceased donors reduces inflammation in the donor liver and improves outcome after liver transplantation: a prospective randomized controlled trial. Ann Surg 2008;248:1042–50.
40. Dimopoulou I, Tsagarakis T, Anthi A, et al. High prevalence of decreased cortisol reserve in brain-dead potential organ donors. Crit Care Med 2003;31:1113–7.
41. Lam L, Inaba K, Branco BC, et al. The impact of early hormonal therapy in catastrophic brain-injured patients and its effect on organ procurement. Am Surg 2012;78:318–24.
42. Schnuelle P, Lorenz D, Muellaer A, et al. Donor catecholamine use reduces acute allograft rejection and improves graft survival after cadaveric renal transplantation. Kidney Int 1999;56:738–46.
43. Gottmann U, Brinkkoetter PT, Bechtler M, et al. Effect of pre-treatment with catecholamines on cold preservation and ischemia/reperfusion-injury in rats. Kidney Int 2006;70:321–8.
44. Mutter TC, Ruth CA, Dart AB. Hydroxyethyl starch (HES) versus other fluid therapies: effects on kidney function. Cochrane Database Syst Rev 2013;(7):CD007594.
45. Myburgh JA, Finfer S, Bellomo R, et al. Hydroxyethyl starch or saline for fluid resuscitation in intensive care. N Engl J Med 2012;367:1901–11.
46. Cittanova ML, Mavre J, Riou B, et al. Long-term follow-up of transplanted kidneys according to plasma volume expander of kidney donors. Intensive Care Med 2001;27:1830.

47. Totsuka E, Dodson F, Urakami A, et al. Influence of high donor serum sodium levels on early postoperative graft function in human liver transplantation: effect of correction of donor hypernatremia. Liver Transpl Surg 1999;5: 421–8.

48. Mangus RS, Fridell JA, Vianna RM, et al. Severe hypernatremia in deceased liver donors does not impact early transplant outcome. Transplantation 2010; 90:438–43.

49. Sato T, Asanuma Y, Yasui O, et al. Impaired hepatic mitochondrial function reserve in brain-dead pigs. Transplant Proc 1998;30:4351–5.

50. Okamoto S, Corso CO, Nolte D, et al. Impact of brain death on hormonal homeostasis and hepatic microcirculation of transplant organ donors. Transpl Int 1998; 11(Suppl 1):S404–407.

51. Compagnon P, Wang H, Lindell SL, et al. Brain death does not affect hepatic allograft function and survival after orthotopic transplantation in a canine model. Transplantation 2002;73:1218–27.

52. Gores PF, Gillingham KJ, Dunn DL, et al. Donor hyperglycemia as a minor risk factor and immunologic variables as major risk factors for pancreas allograft loss in a multivariate analysis of a single institution's experience. Ann Surg 1992;215:217–30.

53. Hefty TR, Cotterell LW, Fraser SC, et al. Disseminated intravascular coagulation in cadaveric organ donors. Incidence and effect on renal transplantation. Transplantation 1993;55:442–3.

54. Hunt SA, Baldwin J, Baumgartner W, et al. Cardiovascular management of a potential heart donor: a statement from the Transplantation Committee of the American College of Cardiology. Crit Care Med 1996;24:1599–601.

55. Wheeldon DR, Potter CD, Oduro A, et al. Transforming the "unacceptable" donor: outcomes from the adoption of a standardized donor management technique. J Heart Lung Transplant 1995;14:734–42.

56. Minambres E, Rodrigo E, Ballesteros MA, et al. Impact of restrictive fluid balance focused to increase lung procurement on renal function after kidney transplantation. Nephrol Dial Transplant 2010;25:2352–6.

57. Abdelnour T, Pieke S. Relationship of hormonal resuscitation therapy and central venous pressure on increasing organs for transplant. J Heart Lung Transplant 2009;28:480–5.

58. Malinoski DJ, Patel MS, Ahmed O, et al. The impact of meeting donor management goals on the development of delayed graft function in kidney transplant recipients. Am J Transplant 2013;13(4):993–1000.

59. Malinoski DJ, Patel MS, Daly MC, et al. The impact of meeting donor management goals on the number of organs transplanted per donor: results from the United Network for Organ Sharing Region 5 prospective donor management goals study. Crit Care Med 2012;40:2773–80.

60. Franklin GA, Santos AP, Smith JW, et al. Optimization of donor management goals yields increased organ use. Am Surg 2010;76:587–94.

61. Hagan ME, McClean D, Falcone CA, et al. Attaining specific donor management goals increases number of organs transplanted per donor: a quality improvement project. Prog Transplant 2009;19:227–31.

62. Malinoski DJ, Daly MC, Patel MS, et al. Achieving donor management goals before deceased donor procurement is associated with more organs transplanted per donor. J Trauma 2011;71:990–5 [discussion: 996].

63. Wetzel RC, Setzer N, Stiff JL. Hemodynamic responses in brain dead organ donor patients. Anesth Analg 1985;64:125–8.

64. Gelb AW, Robertson KM. Anaesthetic management of the brain dead for organ donation. Can J Anaesth 1990;37:806–12.
65. Murugan R, Venkataraman R, Wahed AS, et al. Preload responsiveness is associated with increased interleukin-6 and lower organ yield from brain dead donors. Crit Care Med 2009;37:2387–93.
66. D'Amico F, Vitale A, Piovan D, et al. Use of n-acetylcysteine during liver procurement: a prospective, randomized controlled study. Liver Transpl 2013;19: 135–44.
67. Mone T, Heldens J, Niemann CU. Deceased organ donor research: the last research frontier? Liver Transpl 2013;19:118–21.

Transplantation in ACOs

Zoltan Hevesi, MD, MBA*, Laura Hammel, MD

KEYWORDS

- Health care reform • Medicare • Accountable Care Organization
- Quality improvement • HMO • Patient Centered Medical Home
- Medicare shared savings program

KEY POINTS

- The United States exhibits subpar health care outcomes compared with the Organisation for Economic Co-operation and Development peer group.
- An urgent need exists to address the excessive cost and unsustainable trajectory of expenditures associated with US health care.
- Health care reform ideas based on the Health Maintenance Organization and Patient-Centered Medical Home concepts are a promising solution to address health care inefficiencies.
- Accountable Care Organizations seek to simultaneously improve quality of care and reduce expenditure.

INTRODUCTION

The 20th century is often described as the "American Century," for a good reason. In a political and economic sense, the United States dominated the global stage from the early 1900s and achieved a superpower status after the end of World War II and the subsequent Cold War. By the end of the 20th century, America was often held as the best example of a functioning democracy and racial and religious tolerance, and the most fertile home for innovation.

However, the United States was less successful in the area of health care access, outcome, cost, and efficiency compared with the other similarly developed Organization for Economic Co-operation and Development (OECD) countries. According to the World Health Organization, the United States is trailing its peer group in most outcome and population health metrics, despite spending substantially more per capita than any other nation (**Fig. 1**). In addition, the next 19 wealthiest countries, based on gross domestic product, all gained approximately 6 more years of life expectancy than the

Department of Anesthesiology, University of Wisconsin School of Medicine and Public Health, B6/319 CSC, 600 Highland Avenue, Madison, WI 53792-3272, USA
* Corresponding author.
E-mail address: zghevesi@wisc.edu

Anesthesiology Clin 31 (2013) 749–762
http://dx.doi.org/10.1016/j.anclin.2013.09.003
1932-2275/13/$ – see front matter © 2013 Elsevier Inc. All rights reserved.

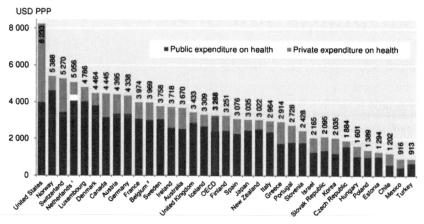

1. In the Netherlands, it is not possible to clearly distinguish the public and private share related to investments.
2. Total expenditure excluding investments.
Information on data for Israel: http://dx.doi.org/10.1787/888932315602.

Fig. 1. The United States spends 2.5 times the OECD average on health care: total health expenditure per capita, public and private, 2010 (or nearest year). (*Courtesy of* The Organisation for Economic Co-operation and Development; with permission. OECD Health Data 2012. Available at: http://www.oecd.org/health/healthdata. Accessed August 29, 2013.)

Americans since 1970 (**Fig. 2**). Furthermore, the prestigious Commonwealth Fund ranked the United States last in the quality of health care among comparable countries.[1–8] Undoubtedly, the United States is different from other nations in many ways: the population is broadly dispersed over a large landmass, which may effect access to health care facilities; obesity is more prevalent; and it has a relatively high

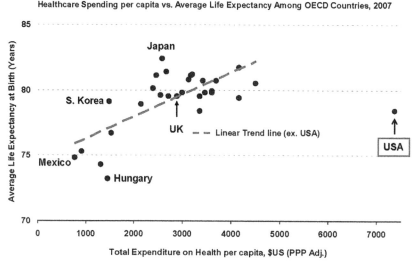

Fig. 2. Life expectancy versus health care spending in 2007. Expenditure in US dollars, corrected for purchasing power parity. (*Data from* Meeker M. USA Inc. KPCB's Web site. Available at: http://www.kpcb.com/insights/2011-usa-inc-full-report. Accessed September 20, 2013.)

murder rate. Nonetheless, the statistics are difficult to explain without a critical look at the health care delivery system.

Most Americans are not acutely concerned with population metrics, and are proud of the ever-improving biotechnology available in the United States. People point out the limitations of the government-run systems, frequently invoking negative examples from the Veterans Administration hospitals or new stories about Great Britain or Canada. Nevertheless, public awareness has been increasing regarding the unsustainable high price of health care and its crippling effects on the country's fiscal health **(Fig. 3)**. Concurrently, some governmental efforts have been made since the 1990s to acknowledge the size of the problem and explore the possible alternatives; however, many of these initial steps fell victim to partisan politics. Health Maintenance Organizations (HMOs) and Patient-Centered Medical Homes (PCMHs) were the 2 most promising concepts of recent health care reform.

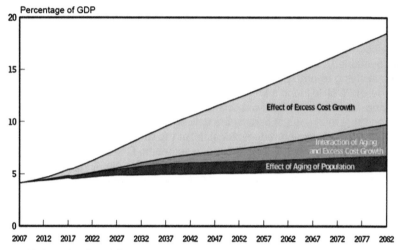

- It is the *rate* of spending per individual that will have the most impact, rather than the *quantity* / demographics of an aging population.
- "Excess cost growth" refers to the extent to which the increase in health care spending for an average individual exceeds the growth in per capita GDP.
- "Interaction..." refers to effects of excess cost growth and the aging of the population, which result in greater growth in spending than would result from either factor separately.
- "Aging of population" refers to demographic shifts, such as an increasing average population age and life expectancy.

Fig. 3. Projected US federal spending on medicare and medicaid as a percentage of gross domestic product (GDP). (*From* Congressional budget office. Health care: capturing the opportunity in the nation's core fiscal challenge. Available at: http://cbo.gov/sites/default/files/cbofiles/ftpdocs/90xx/doc9054/03-12-princetonwnews.pdf.)

HMOS

Early forms of prepaid health plans existed in the United States as early as the 1910s. The Ross-Loos Medical Group (established in 1929) is considered the first classic large-scale HMO, providing a broad spectrum of health services for more than 30,000 Los Angeles public employees by the 1950s. This HMO, after a series of mergers and acquisition, became known as CIGNA. Similarly, the origins of Blue Cross can be traced back to 1929 when Baylor Hospital offered a prepaid health plan for 1500 teachers. HMOs grew rapidly during the Great Depression, offering a steady cash flow for health care providers.

By the 1970s, the popularity of HMOs declined and the number of these organizations decreased dramatically. To curb the rate of medical cost inflation, President

Richard Nixon signed the Health Maintenance Organization Act of 1973, which is also known as the Federal HMO Act.[9,10] The law included the Dual Choice mandate: employers with 25 or more employees who offered traditional health insurance coverage were required to also offer a federally certified HMO option.[11]

Ultimately, however, federal certification and grant support were not entirely successful in saving the reputation of HMOs from the criticism of compromised access and quality of care while maintaining the primary focus on cost reduction. Additionally, the public was often appalled to learn about the high administrative costs and very generous executive compensation in contrast to the frugality experienced by the subscribers.

PCMHS

The term *medical home* was introduced by the American Academy of Pediatrics in 1967. The concept envisioned a continuous and coordinated care for children, especially those with special needs.[12,13] After decades of gradual evolution, in 2002, the concept became the centerpiece of the Future of Family Medicine project, a joint venture of 7 national family medicine organizations advocating for a care that was "accessible, accountable, comprehensive, integrated, patient-centered, safe, scientifically valid and satisfying to both patients and their physicians."[14]

The model of PCMHs found many supporters in consumer groups, large employers, insurers, and numerous medical associations.[15,16] A variety of pilot programs and studies found that this mode of health care delivery resulted in improved access, better overall quality of care, and reduced cost, all at the same time.[17] The Accreditation Association for Ambulatory Health Care began accrediting medical homes in 2009 as the only accrediting body conducting on-site surveys. The *New England Journal of Medicine* endorsed the PCMH concept in 2008, and recommended increased information sharing between care providers, broadening of the performance measures, and shared cost savings with physicians as opportunities for improvement.[18] By 2009, 10 states introduced a total of 20 bills supporting the establishment of medical homes.[19]

PATIENT PROTECTION AND AFFORDABLE CARE ACT OF 2010

Most Americans agree for one reason or another that the current US health care system must be improved. For some, it is the lack of universal access that provides justification for change; for others, it is the high and rapidly growing cost; and for yet others, it is the often futile wasteful care. The national dialogue about the main guiding principles and the desirable direction of the change is where the people's consensus stops and tremendous anxiety begins; this has been on full display ever since the 2008 presidential election.

After much bipartisan fighting, President Barack Obama signed into law the Patient Protection and Affordable Care Act (PPACA; Public Law 111–148), the product of the Democratic 111th Congress and the White House, on March 23, 2010. The provisions spelled out in the law are scheduled to take effect via gradual implementation over 4 years. The PPACA includes a large number of complex and drastic changes from the baseline, such as a much expanded Medicaid program, subsidized and capped insurance premiums for a large segment of the population, protection for patients with preexisting medical conditions, and establishment of insurance exchanges. The costs of these ambitious provisions are offset by a variety of taxes and fees. The net effect of the PPACA and the Health Care and Education Reconciliation Act of 2010 combined is estimated by the Congressional Budget Office to produce a cost reduction of $143 billion over a decade; this figure is vehemently contested by the opponents of this law. The critics assert that improved care coordination and government-enforced quality control cannot trim down expenditures in the face of continued indiscriminate overconsumption of health care services by a large population that is sheltered from the costs via government subsidies.

ACCOUNTABLE CARE ORGANIZATIONS

The term *Accountable Care Organization* was first used in 2006 during a public meeting of the Medicare Payment Advisory Commission and was later included in the PPACA of 2010.[20] The ACO model bears much resemblance to the essence of HMOs, and builds on 2 recent successful prototypes by Kaiser Permanente and HealthCare Partner Medical Groups. The 3 main principles are as follows:

1. Provider-led organizations with a strong base of primary care that are collectively accountable for quality and total per capita costs across the full continuum of care for a population of patients;
2. Payments linked to quality improvements that also reduce overall costs; and,
3. Reliable and progressively more sophisticated performance measurement to support improvement and provide confidence that savings are achieved through improvements in care.[21]

While allowing patients complete freedom to choose from the available medical service providers, the ACO model places the responsibility on the health care organizations to improve quality of care and reduce expenditure simultaneously. This goal is to be achieved by fostering highly coordinated and data-driven evidence-based practices. Unfortunately, at the time of writing, a substantial uncertainty exists about the details of implementation, minimum criteria for participation for organizations, typical amount of investment for successful operation, national quality benchmarks, and the specific savings goals, to name just the major concerns.

ACOS: WHAT IS KNOWN?

The ACO model was included in the national health care reform as one of several programs to be administered by the Center for Medicare and Medicaid Services (CMS), along with bundled payments and other novel approaches. Section 3022 of the PPACA authorized the CMS to launch a Medicare Shared Savings Program (MSSP) and offer ACO contracting with Medicare from January of 2012.[22] In the MSSP, the ACO assumes the care of a defined group of Medicare Fee-For-Services beneficiaries, including the overall quality and cost for a duration of 3 years.

The details of the ACO contracts were left to the judgment of the Secretary of the Department of Health and Human Services (DHHS).[23] To be eligible for the ACO designation and entering into an ACO contract with Medicare, the candidate health care organization must fulfill several strictly defined requirements as defined by the DHHS final rule (October 20, 2011)[24]:

- The ACO shall be willing to become accountable for the quality, cost, and overall care of the Medicare Fee-For-Service beneficiaries assigned to it.
- The ACO shall enter into an agreement with the Secretary to participate in the program for not less than a 3-year period.
- The ACO shall have a formal legal structure that would allow the organization to receive and distribute payments for shared savings to participating providers of services and suppliers.

- The ACO shall include primary care ACO professionals that are sufficient for the number of Medicare Fee-For-Service beneficiaries assigned to the ACO under subsection.
- At a minimum, the ACO shall have at least 5000 of these beneficiaries assigned to it to be eligible to participate in the ACO program.
- The ACO shall provide the Secretary with this information regarding ACO professionals participating in the ACO, because the Secretary determines necessary to support the assignment of Medicare Fee-For-Service beneficiaries to an ACO, the implementation of quality and other reporting requirements under paragraph (3), and the determination of payments for shared savings under subsection (d)(2).
- The ACO shall have in place a leadership and management structure that includes clinical and administrative systems.
- The ACO shall define processes to promote evidence-based medicine and patient engagement, report on quality and cost measures, and coordinate care, such as through the use of telehealth, remote patient monitoring, and other enabling technologies.
- The ACO shall demonstrate to the Secretary that it meets patient-centeredness criteria specified by the Secretary, such as the use of patient and caregiver assessments or the use of individualized care plans.
- The ACO participant cannot participate in other Medicare shared savings programs.
- The ACO entity is responsible for distributing savings to participating entities.
- The ACO must have a process for evaluating the health needs of the population it serves.[25]

Moreover, according to the final regulations released by the DHHS, the ACO must chose from 2 payment models—1-sided versus 2-sided—based on the level of its risk tolerance. The amount of the assumed risk determines the level of participation of the potential savings. In the 1-sided model, the bonus payment is a predetermined percentage of the difference between the organization's annual expenditure and the CMS benchmark minus a 2% minimum savings; and the ACO assumes no financial risk. In the 2-sided model, the providers assume a preset level of financial risk if the cost of care exceeds the CMS benchmarks; however, they have a potential to earn a larger portion of the savings without the 2% minimum saving subtracted from the benchmark.

Having learned from the HMO experiences, to assure that the health care providers' cost reduction is not achieved by limiting patient access and/or compromising quality of care, the ACO's performance is monitored by a set of 33 quality measures in 4 domains (**Box 1**).[26] Meeting the quality goals serves as the minimal criterion for participating in any of the financial incentive payments and shared savings. The American Hospital Association expressed concern related to the high startup cost, large annual maintenance expenses, and the lack of specific information about the ACO implementation in 2011.[27]

PAST PILOT PROGRAMS AND ONGOING INITIATIVES

ACO-like payment and delivery models have been tested since 1998, and a limited amount of research on their findings has been published. The most notable examples are the Community Care of North Carolina (1998), the Physician Group Practice Demonstration (2005), and the Pathways to Health initiative of Battle Creek, Michigan (2006).[21,28,29] These programs were combinations of federal, state, and local projects

---

Box 1
Quality measures in 4 domains to monitor quality of care

- Patient/caregiver experience (7 measures)
- Care coordination/patient safety (6 measures)
- Preventive health (8 measures)
- At-risk population:

  Diabetes (1 measure and 1 composite consisting of 5 measures)

  Hypertension (1 measure)

  Ischemic vascular disease (2 measures)

  Heart failure (1 measure)

  Coronary artery disease (1 composite consisting of 2 measures)

---

that shared some of the key characteristics of the ACO model, such as the alignment of incentives among patients, payers, and a diverse array of providers. These ventures substantiated the benefits of care coordination and evidence-based clinical practices: the quality improvements and cost reductions.

Current federal and private programs may further elucidate the specific methods to achieve the intended targets of the ACO model. The Brookings-Dartmouth Accountable Care Collaborative and the Robert Wood Johnson Foundation Medical School projects are focusing on the shared incentives and local accountability features of the ACOs; the Baylor Health System program is testing of different bundled payment systems; and the Premier ACO Collaborative is examining the various aspects of successful ACO implementation.[30]

NATIONAL SURVEY OF HOSPITAL READINESS TO PARTICIPATE IN AN ACO

As of late 2011, only 13% of hospitals participated or planned to participate in ACOs within a year. In contrast, 75% had no intention of participating in ACOs at all.[31] Typically, the participating or planning-to-participate hospitals consisted of large teaching and nonprofit organizations, belonged to a health system, and were located in larger urban areas. These numbers clearly indicate that the ACO adoption process is in its early stages.

In terms of governance of the ACO participants and planning-to-participate organizations, 51% were joint ventures between hospitals and physicians and 18% were physician-led groups (**Fig. 4**). Most respondents were expecting a significant decrease in revenue from fee-for-service payments while hoping for an increase from bundled and shared savings. Most hospitals (52.1%) reported pursuing the 1-sided shared savings ACO model that did not expose them to potential financial loss (**Fig. 5**). This finding confirms the logic that management infrastructure and care coordination must be present before an organization should assume the financial risk involved in caring for a defined patient population. Moreover, the results of the survey clearly indicate that many hospitals did not have the comprehensive quality and cost monitoring programs essential for the ACO approach.

A more recent survey identified 221 CMS and private sector ACOs in 45 states as of May of 2012.[32] The most frequently identified challenges to ACO participations were reducing clinical care variations, reducing cost of care, and developing a common culture among ACO partners. The CMS innovation center offers a pioneer ACO program

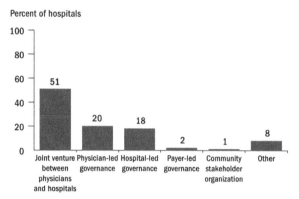

Fig. 4. Governance of hospitals participating or planning to participate in an ACO (n = 182). (*From* Audet AM, Kenward K, Patel S, et al. Hospitals on the path to accountable care: highlights from a 2011 national survey of hospital readiness to participate in an accountable care organization. Issue Brief (Commonwealth Fund) 2012;22:1–12.)

to promote and sustain the next wave of improvements coming from strong organizations with a potential to advance the ACO model. Simultaneously, the DHHS offers an array of alternative options and incentives, including bundled payments for care improvement and a community-based transitional care program, for other organizations that are not ready to transition into an ACO yet.

ORGAN TRANSPLANTATION AND THE ACO APPROACH

The Organ Procurement and Transplant Network (OPTN) was created by the US Congress in 1984 to oversee the fair distribution of the critically limited resource of transplantable organs (**Figs. 6** and **7**). In collaboration with the nonprofit United Network for Organ Sharing, these organizations provide a great example of the effectiveness of data-driven and evidence-based medical management. The once-subjective process of organ transplant candidate selection and prioritization was

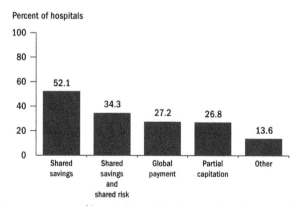

Fig. 5. Payment arrangements of hospitals participating or planning to participate in an ACO (n = 213). (*From* Audet AM, Kenward K, Patel S, et al. Hospitals on the path to accountable care: highlights from a 2011 national survey of hospital readiness to participate in an accountable care organization. Issue Brief (Commonwealth Fund) 2012;22:1–12.)

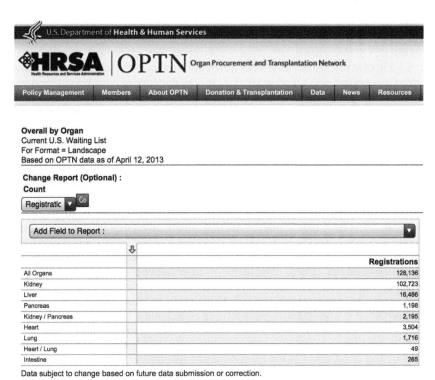

Fig. 6. OPTN waiting list for organ transplantation, April 2013. (*From* U.S. Department of Health and Human Services. Organ Procurement and Transplantation Network Database. Available at: http://optn.transplant.hrsa.gov/data/.)

transformed into an objective process over the past 25 years, improving fairness and saving countless lives along the way. Organ transplantation became the preferred treatment for a rapidly growing list of medical conditions, and the number of transplanted organs increased steadily.

At the time of writing, more than 128,000 patients are waiting for various organ transplantations, according to the OPTN. This waiting list has been steadily growing

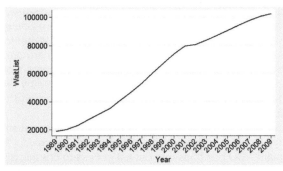

Fig. 7. OPTN waiting list growth since 1989. (*From* U.S. Department of Health and Human Services. Organ Procurement and Transplantation Network Database. Available at: http://optn.transplant.hrsa.gov.)

every year ever since the OPTN was established. Patients with single or multiple organ failure represent a small fraction of the Medicare population and a disproportionately higher fraction of Medicare expenditure. For example, end-stage renal disease (ESRD) affects 1.3% of Medicare recipients but accounts for approximately 7.5% of Medicare spending, exceeding $20 billion in 2010. Similarly, patients with liver, lung, and heart failure present significant therapeutic complexity, a predisposition for multiple comorbidities, and a greatly increased potential for an endless list of possibly devastating and pricey complications. Because of these intricate and disproportionally expensive medical conditions, a high potential for quality improvement and cost savings exists through optimizing medical care delivery for these patients.

Organ transplantation and the associated perioperative medical care made tremendous strides in the last half century. Although better immune therapy was probably the main factor in this success story, the improved understanding of pathomechanisms, countless innovations (medical, surgical, biotechnological), and enhanced donor management all undeniably contributed to the much-increased long-term survival rates of the organ transplant recipients. However, despite the extraordinary advances, further opportunities clearly exist for optimizing outcome and reducing the use of resources. Immense variability of clinical care seems to exist between transplantation centers, and best practices that are based on available published medical evidence are often implemented after considerable delay.[33] Much remains to be gained from improved information sharing and attentive medical care coordination between various collaborating medical specialties, as opposed to the current system that is more fittingly described as *parallel processing*. The ideal system must support the accumulation of training and experience in the form of highly specialized teams but, at the same time, prevent the evolution of isolated silos.[34] Sensitive balancing of these seemingly contradicting imperatives requires mindful organizational development, collaborative culture, appropriately aligned system of incentives, and engaged leadership.

In addition to the known challenges of ACO implementation, the field of organ transplantation presents a set of special considerations not usually associated with other medical care. When examining patient survival and cost of care, for instance, organ transplantation surgery involves a large initial investment, both in terms of human capital and material resources, and the benefits of improved quality of life and increased life expectancy do not materialize directly after surgery. In fact, in the immediate postoperative period, survival expectation is temporarily reduced because of the possibility of perioperative complications. Furthermore, although risk-adjusted 1-, 3-, and 5-year graft and patient survivals are well-established benchmarks when comparing various transplantation centers or historical periods, and an abundance of data have been collected by OPTN over decades, it is challenging to set ACO benchmarks for quality metrics and cost expectations that allow a Medicare Shared Savings Program to be implemented. Comparing various outcome and cost metrics is only meaningful if they are sensitive to the differences per phases of care and adjust for the variability described earlier. Moreover, median waiting time, percent of listed patients transplanted, and waiting list mortality rates are highly variable by region and organ transplantation center, and some of these metrics are far beyond the control and influence of the transplantation programs.

In addition to observable outcome and cost-of-care metrics, patient and caregiver experience surveys must be included in the evaluation of successful ACO implementation. The transplant ACO has to assure patient access to chronic disease management, sophisticated monitoring of organ functions, bridge therapies (eg, dialysis, ventricular assist devices), organ transplantation surgeries, and postoperative care, which includes the possibility of retransplantation if necessary. Currently, in the pre-ACO environment, many transplant candidates have specialists (eg, nephrologists, hepatologists, cardiologists, pulmonologists) functioning as primary care physicians to oversee the complex medical management. This dynamic is somewhat of an anomaly compared with the ACO vision, which promotes the importance of primary care physicians as the best positioned to coordinate overall care.

In February of 2013, the CMS released some details for a newly created renal ACO demonstration, called ESRD Seamless Care Organization (ESCO).[35] A few specifics are currently known about ESCO beyond the generic ACO criteria and guiding principles. The deadline for application is May, 2013. In the area of reimbursement, CMS introduced a new model for cost benchmarking that involves "historical matching" and "quarterly matching," a look-back approach to assess medical spending. According to the plan, when evaluating the average per-capita expenditure for each performance year, the historical expenditure baseline will be risk-adjusted, trended, price-adjusted, and bundle-adjusted to form an updated benchmark. Three different payment tracks were created: 1 for ESCOs with a large dialysis center and a choice between 2 other tracks for ESCOs without a large dialysis facility. All 3 tracks are 2-sided, involving both savings potential and financial risk sharing by the second and third year of the ACO contract, and the minimal savings rate is set between 1% and 4% based on the payment track and the size of the patient population.

How other organ transplantations will evolve as the health care reform is gradually implemented remains to be seen. It is conceivable that cardiovascular disease, a major contributor to morbidity and mortality, will be appropriate for the ACO model, similar to the ESCO demonstration for ESRD care. Obviously in this scenario, heart transplantation would be a small fraction of the many activities that such a cardiovascular-focused ACO center would cover. Lung, liver, and pancreas transplantation, all with a much smaller number of transplantation candidates and surgeries per year compared with renal transplantation, may not be practical to organize according to the ACO model. Other approaches, such as a combination of predefined quality metrics and bundled payments, may prove to be more effective to incentivize comprehensive high-quality and reduced-cost care. Success or failure of the early ACO programs will have much to do with shaping the future of health care development.

KEY QUESTIONS TO CONSIDER AND NEXT STEPS FOR ACOS

The main driving forces for health care reform and the key principles of the ACO concept are difficult to dispute. The implementation will determine the long-term impact and viability of this ambitious plan. The ACO idea is the latest of several endeavors to improve the US medical system; in large part, it is based on the HMO and PCMH experiences. Building on the strengths and correcting the weaknesses of previous attempts is a rational start, but it does not eliminate unintended consequences. The more policy advisers and health care leaders anticipate and address the potential challenges, the better are the chances of the ACO ventures.

Improved awareness about the current status and unsustainable trajectory of Medicare is paramount to gain acceptance of the necessary adjustments. Anxiety over the anticipated changes often leads to political maneuvering and eventual inaction. The longer the inevitable is delayed, the fewer feasible options will be available. An educated and engaged public is perhaps the most fundamental element of success in this scenario. Similarly, US physicians (>850,000 individuals per the 2010 census) and other health care professionals present powerful intellectual and political strengths that may become formidable forces in support of, or against, this particular reorganization model. Detailed explanation of the rationales and the action plan will significantly help secure professional support for the intended transformation. To eliminate physician barriers to integration, crucial elements such as the setting of quality benchmarks and the formulae for savings calculations must be clearly communicated.

The optimal size of the ACO presents an interesting dilemma for hospital and health plan administrators: on one hand, consolidation into a large organization makes sense to make large investments in the necessary ACO infrastructure reasonable and profitable; however, on the other hand, redistribution of shared Medicare incentives is increasingly more complex the larger an institution gets. To achieve optimal economy of scale, minimum annual revenue in the range of $5 billion to $50 billion is often quoted, a huge sum when contrasted with today's typical establishments.

Last but not least, much concern exists on the part of future ACO candidate organizations regarding the regulatory environment. Market consolidation for the purpose of ACO formation and institutionalized redistribution of the incentives generated from MSSP are potential violations of the Sherman Act of 1890, the gold standard antitrust statute in US law.[36] In October 2011, the Federal Trade Commission and the Department of Justice issued the Statement of Antitrust Enforcement Policy Regarding Accountable Care Organizations participating in the Medicare Shared Savings Program to clarify the law, and offered an expedited 90-day review for organizations contemplating ACO formation. Some questions remain concerning the antitrust issues regarding the definition of the local market and the size of the health care entities interested in becoming an ACO.

SUMMARY

The early 21st century is proving to be an interesting time. There exists an urgent need to correct the unsustainable trajectory of US health care costs and a simultaneous pressure to elevate outcomes to the level of other developed OECD member countries.

ACOs are just one of the proposed ways to achieve the stated goals; it is a well-intended concept but has no proven track record on the national scale. Constructive participation in overcoming the challenges will determine how physicians will be viewed by the rest of the citizenry and the future.

REFERENCES

1. World Health Organization. World Health Statistics 2009. Available at: http://www.who.int/whosis/whostat/2009/en/. Accessed September 5, 2013.
2. World Health Organization. World Health Statistics 2011. Available at: http://www.who.int/whosis/whostat/2011/en/. Accessed September 5, 2013.
3. Anderson GF, Reinhardt UE, Hussey PS, et al. It's the prices, stupid: why the United States is so different from other countries. Health Aff (Millwood) 2003; 22(3):89–105.
4. Roehr B. Health care in US ranks lowest among developed countries. BMJ 2008; 337:a889.
5. Davis K, Schoen C, Stremikis K. Mirror, mirror on the wall: how the performance of the U.S. health care system compares internationally. 2010 Update. Available at: http://www.commonwealthfund.org/~/media/Files/Publications/Fund%20Report/2010/Jun/1400_Davis_Mirror_Mirror_on_the_wall_2010.pdf. Accessed September 5, 2013.
6. Available at: https://www.cia.gov/library/publications/the-world-factbook/rankorder/2102rank.html?countryName=United%20States&;countryCode=us&regionCode=noa&rank=50#us.

7. Wilper AP, Woolhandler S, Lasser KE, et al. Health insurance and mortality in US adults. Am J Public Health 2009;99(12):2289–95.
8. Hadley J. Insurance coverage, medical care use, and short-term health changes following an unintentional injury or the onset of a chronic condition. JAMA 2007; 297:1073–84.
9. Rosoff AJ. The Federal HMO Assistance Act: Helping Hand or Hurdle? American Business Law Journal 1975;13(2):137.
10. Patel K, Rushefsky M. Health care politics and policy in America. 3rd edition. Armonk (NY): M.E. Sharpe; 2006.
11. Thrower E, Manders JM. Legislated market access: the historical and legislative evolution of the dual choice mandate in the federal HMO act. J Insur Regul 1988; 7(2):191.
12. Sia C, Tonniges TF, Osterhus E, et al. History of the medical home concept. Pediatrics 2004;113(Suppl 5):1473–8.
13. American Academy of Pediatrics Ad Hoc Task Force on Definition of the Medical Home: the medical home. Pediatrics 1992;90(5):774.
14. Martin JC, Avant RF, Bowman MA, et al. The future of family medicine: a collaborative project of the family medicine community. Ann Fam Med 2004;2(Suppl 1): S3–32.
15. Backer LA. Building the case for the patient-centered medical home. Fam Pract Manag 2009;16(1):14–8.
16. American Academy of Family Physicians. Joint principles of the patient-centered medical home. Del Med J 2008;80(1):21–2.
17. Homer CJ, Klatka K, Romm D, et al. A review of the evidence for the medical home for children with special health care needs. Pediatrics 2008;122(4): e922–37.
18. Fisher ES. Building a medical neighborhood for the medical home. N Engl J Med 2008;359(12):1202–5.
19. Rittenhouse DR, Shortell SM. The patient-centered medical home: will it stand the test of health reform? J Am Med Assoc 2009;301(19):2038–40.
20. Fisher ES, Staiger DO, Bynum J, et al. Creating accountable care organizations: the extended hospital medical staff. Health Aff (Millwood) 2007;26(1): w44–57.
21. McClellan M, McKethan AN, Lewis JL, et al. A national strategy to put accountable care into practice. Health Aff (Millwood) 2010;29(5):982–90.
22. Gold J. Accountable Care Organizations, explained. NPR Web site. Available at: http://www.npr.org/2011/04/01/132937232/accountable-care-organizations-explained. Accessed September 5, 2013.
23. Accountable Care Organizations: what providers need to know. Department of Health and Human Services: Centers for Medicare & Medicaid Services Web site. Available at: http://www.cms.gov/Medicare/Medicare-Fee-for-Service-Payment/sharedsavingsprogram/Downloads/ACO_Providers_Factsheet_ ICN907406.pdf. Accessed September 5, 2013.
24. Berwick DM. Making good on ACOs' promise—the final rule for the medicare shared savings program. N Engl J Med 2011;365:1753–6.
25. Shared savings program. Centers for Medicare & Medicaid Services Web site. Available at: https://www.cms.gov/sharedsavingsprogram/. Accessed September 5, 2013.
26. Centers for Medicare & Medicaid Services (CMS), HHS. Medicare program; Medicare Shared Savings Program: Accountable Care Organizations. Final rule. Fed Regist 2011;76(212):67802–990.

27. The work ahead: activities and costs to develop an accountable care organization. American Hospital Association Web site. Available at: http://www.aha.org/content/11/aco-white-paper-cost-dev-aco.pdf. Accessed September 5, 2013.

28. Community Care of North Carolina: putting health reform ideas into practice in Medicaid. The Henry J. Kaiser Family Foundation Web site. Available at: http://kff.org/health-reform/issue-brief/community-care-of-north-carolina-putting-health/. Accessed September 5, 2013.

29. Simmons J. The medical home as community effort. Health Leaders April 2010. p. 50–1.

30. Accountable Care Organizations: a new model for sustainable innovation. Deloitte Web site. Available at: http://www.deloitte.com/assets/Dcom-UnitedStates/Local%20Assets/Documents/US_CHS_AccountableCareOrganizations_070610.pdf. Accessed September 5, 2013.

31. Hospital readiness for population-based accountable care. Hospitals in Pursuit of Excellence Web site. Available at: http://www.hpoe.org/resources/hpoehretaha-guides/804. Accessed September 5, 2013.

32. Muhlestein D, Croshaw A, Merrill T, et al. Growth and dispersion of Accountable Care Organizations. Available at: http://leavittpartners.com/wp-content/uploads/2013/03/Growth-and-Dispersion-of-ACOs-June-2012-Update-Download.pdf. Accessed September 5, 2013.

33. Schuman R. Intraoperative resource utilization in anesthesia for liver transplantation in the United States: a survey. Anesth Analg 2003;97:21–8.

34. Hevesi ZG, Lopukhin SY, Mezrich JD, et al. Designated liver transplant anesthesia team reduces blood transfusion, need for mechanical ventilation, and duration of intensive care. Liver Transpl 2009;15:460–5.

35. Comprehensive ESRD Care Initiative. Centers for Medicare & Medicaid Services Web site. Available at: http://innovation.cms.gov/initiatives/comprehensive-ESRD-care/. Accessed September 5, 2013.

36. Sherman Act. Public L No. 94-435, 3 §305(a), 90 Stat 1383.

Index

Note: Page numbers of article titles are in **boldface** type.

Anesthesiology Clin 31 (2013) 763–770
http://dx.doi.org/10.1016/S1932-2275(13)00092-X
1932-2275/13/$ – see front matter © 2013 Elsevier Inc. All rights reserved.
                anesthesiology.theclinics.com

United States Postal Service

Statement of Ownership, Management, and Circulation
(All Periodicals Publications Except Requestor Publications)

1. Publication Title	2. Publication Number	3. Filing Date
Anesthesiology Clinics	0 0 0 - 2 7 7 7	9/14/13

4. Issue Frequency	5. Number of Issues Published Annually	6. Annual Subscription Price
Mar, Jun, Sep, Dec	4	$313.00

7. Complete Mailing Address of Known Office of Publication (Not printer) (Street, city, county, state, and ZIP+4®)

Elsevier Inc.
360 Park Avenue South
New York, NY 10010-1710

Contact Person: Stephen R. Bushing
Telephone (Include area code): 215-239-3688

8. Complete Mailing Address of Headquarters or General Business Office of Publisher (Not printer)

Elsevier Inc., 360 Park Avenue South, New York, NY 10010-1710

9. Full Names and Complete Mailing Addresses of Publisher, Editor, and Managing Editor (Do not leave blank)

Publisher (Name and complete mailing address)

Linda Belfus, Elsevier, Inc., 1600 John F. Kennedy Blvd. Suite 1800, Philadelphia, PA 19103-2899

Editor (Name and complete mailing address)

Pamela Hetherington, Elsevier, Inc., 1600 John F. Kennedy Blvd. Suite 1800, Philadelphia, PA 19103-2899

Managing Editor (Name and complete mailing address)

Adrianne Brigido, Elsevier, Inc., 1600 John F. Kennedy Blvd. Suite 1800, Philadelphia, PA 19103-2899

10. Owner (Do not leave blank. If the publication is owned by a corporation, give the name and address of the corporation immediately followed by the names and addresses of all stockholders owning or holding 1 percent or more of the total amount of stock. If not owned by a corporation, give the names and addresses of the individual owners. If owned by a partnership or other unincorporated firm, give its name and address as well as those of each individual owner. If the publication is published by a nonprofit organization, give its name and address.)

Full Name	Complete Mailing Address
Wholly owned subsidiary of	1600 John F. Kennedy Blvd., Ste. 1800
Reed/Elsevier, US holdings	Philadelphia, PA 19103-2899

11. Known Bondholders, Mortgagees, and Other Security Holders Owning or Holding 1 Percent or More of Total Amount of Bonds, Mortgages, or Other Securities. If none, check box ☐ None

Full Name	Complete Mailing Address
N/A	

12. Tax Status (For completion by nonprofit organizations authorized to mail at nonprofit rates) (Check one)
The purpose, function, and nonprofit status of this organization and the exempt status for federal income tax purposes:
☐ Has Not Changed During Preceding 12 Months
☐ Has Changed During Preceding 12 Months (Publisher must submit explanation of change with this statement)

PS Form 3526, September 2007 (Page 1 of 3 (Instructions Page 3)) PSN 7530-01-000-9931 PRIVACY NOTICE: See our Privacy policy in www.usps.com

---

13. Publication Title	14. Issue Date for Circulation Data Below
Anesthesiology Clinics	September 2013

15. Extent and Nature of Circulation			Average No. Copies Each Issue During Preceding 12 Months	No. Copies of Single Issue Published Nearest to Filing Date
a. Total Number of Copies (Net press run)			809	972
b. Paid Circulation (By Mail and Outside the Mail)	(1)	Mailed Outside-County Paid Subscriptions Stated on PS Form 3541. (Include paid distribution above nominal rate, advertiser's proof copies, and exchange copies)	346	469
	(2)	Mailed In-County Paid Subscriptions Stated on PS Form 3541 (Include paid distribution above nominal rate, advertiser's proof copies, and exchange copies)		
	(3)	Paid Distribution Outside the Mails Including Sales Through Dealers and Carriers, Street Vendors, Counter Sales, and Other Paid Distribution Outside USPS®	195	252
	(4)	Paid Distribution by Other Classes Mailed Through the USPS (e.g. First-Class Mail®)		
c. Total Paid Distribution (Sum of 15b (1), (2), (3), and (4))			541	721
d. Free or Nominal Rate Distribution (By Mail and Outside the Mail)	(1)	Free or Nominal Rate Outside-County Copies Included on PS Form 3541	92	111
	(2)	Free or Nominal Rate In-County Copies Included on PS Form 3541		
	(3)	Free or Nominal Rate Copies Mailed at Other Classes Through the USPS (e.g. First-Class Mail)		
	(4)	Free or Nominal Rate Distribution Outside the Mail (Carriers or other means)		
e. Total Free or Nominal Rate Distribution (Sum of 15d (1), (2), (3) and (4))			92	111
f. Total Distribution (Sum of 15c and 15e)			633	832
g. Copies not Distributed (See instructions to publishers #4 (page #3))			176	140
h. Total (Sum of 15f and g)			809	972
i. Percent Paid (15c divided by 15f times 100)			85.47%	86.66%

16. Publication of Statement of Ownership

☐ If the publication is a general publication, publication of this statement is required. Will be printed in the December 2013 issue of this publication.   ☐ Publication not required

17. Signature and Title of Editor, Publisher, Business Manager, or Owner

[signature] Stephen R. Bushing

Stephen R. Bushing – Inventory Distribution Coordinator

Date: September 14, 2013

I certify that all information furnished on this form is true and complete. I understand that anyone who furnishes false or misleading information on this form or who omits material or information requested on the form may be subject to criminal sanctions (including fines and imprisonment) and/or civil sanctions (including civil penalties).

PS Form 3526, September 2007 (Page 2 of 3)

Moving?

Make sure your subscription moves with you!

To notify us of your new address, find your **Clinics Account Number** (located on your mailing label above your name), and contact customer service at:

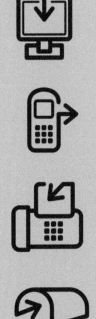

Email: journalscustomerservice-usa@elsevier.com

800-654-2452 (subscribers in the U.S. & Canada)
314-447-8871 (subscribers outside of the U.S. & Canada)

Fax number: 314-447-8029

Elsevier Health Sciences Division
Subscription Customer Service
3251 Riverport Lane
Maryland Heights, MO 63043

ELSEVIER

Printed and bound by CPI Group (UK) Ltd, Croydon, CR0 4YY

03/10/2024

01040493-0012